# Losing It!

# Losing It!

## An LDS Guide to Healthy Living

**Melanie Douglass**

**Registered Dietitian**
**NASM Certified Personal Trainer**

**ICON Health & Fitness**

DESERET
BOOK

SALT LAKE CITY, UTAH

To my husband, Danny, and our children,

Abbi, Britley, and Tavan, for bringing happiness and harmony to my life.

You make me want to be a healthier person.

The advice and recommendations presented in this book are intended as an educational resource to assist readers in making informed decisions. This book is not intended to replace the advice of a medical professional. Always seek the advice of your physician before beginning this or any exercise and nutrition program. The author and publisher disclaim any liability arising from directly or indirectly using this book.

**Library of Congress Cataloging-in-Publication Data**

Douglass, Melanie.
  Losing it! / Melanie Douglass.
    p.  cm.
  Includes bibliographical references and index.
  ISBN 1-59038-430-X (pbk.)
  1. Weight loss—Religious aspects—Church of Jesus Christ of Latter-day Saints.  I. Title.
  RM222.2.D6763  2005
  613.2'5—dc22                                           2005013653

Printed in the United States of America         72076
Publishers Printing, Salt Lake City, UT

10  9   8   7   6   5   4   3   2   1

# Contents

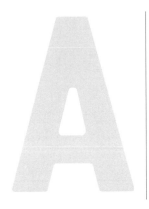# Acknowledgments

With genuine gratitude and appreciation to:

My parents, Van and Marsha, and my in-laws, Paul and Jean, for their unwavering love and support for me, my husband, and my precious children. I don't know where I would be without you.

Cathy Chamberlain, Jana Erickson, and Sheri Dew, my friends and supporters at Deseret Book, for asking me to write this book and for their strong belief in the message of good health. Your valuable insight helped me capture the right message for this book.

Scott Watterson, founder of ICON Health & Fitness, for believing in me. The impact of your creativity, perseverance, and sense of purpose in the health industry is beyond measure.

And lastly, my colleagues at ICON Health & Fitness, an amazing company with genuinely good people and remarkable products that change lives by offering something we all need: vitality, strength, and lifelong health.

# Introduction

*Losing it.* In any other facet of our lives, "losing it" can be a bad thing. When it comes to being overweight, "losing it" is nothing but good. Improved health, for anyone who lives and breathes in America today, comes from building habits that originate from the "losing it" mindset. It may be losing weight, losing excess body fat, losing the daily morning donut, losing negative thoughts about the way our bodies look, or even losing a few precious minutes of each day to exercise.

As obesity rates have soared over the past few years, I've watched, pained, as food has become the enemy, exercise has become the punishment, and happiness—as related to body image—has become the unattainable. Many people feel stuck in an unhealthy society that is obsessed with weight. The weight-loss products and services industry rakes in more than $33 billion dollars every year in the United States.[1] Sadly, the massive amount of money we spend on "improving our lives" has not seemed to help the 65 percent of American adults who are now overweight.[2] Most of us have thrown in the towel—we are sick of no-carb, high-carb, low-fat, high-fat, high-protein, grapefruit-juice, cabbage-soup, and all the other "diet" diets. We are sick of exercise advice that changes by the day.

Additionally, few of us seem to understand what "good health" even is anymore. The media would have us believe that good health is about restriction, punishment, and manipulation of our bodies. Marketing and advertising agencies would have us believe that good health is all about body weight—the perfect size. Maybe the problem isn't our weight at all. Maybe the problem is about how we live day to day. In the end, good health is just that—a lifestyle that promotes a sound mind, body, and spirit and that is free from physical pain and disease. Whether nine or ninety years old, underweight or obese, athletic or couch potato, we all need to move more and make better eating choices in order to become healthy.

Think about three words for a moment: *food, exercise,* and *health.* How many of us are affected by these highly interconnected words every day? Sometimes "exercise" and "health" don't make our daily priority list, but every day each one of us is affected by food. As humans, we have always been intimately connected with food. Day after day, we devote precious hours to acquiring, storing, preparing, cooking, serving, eating, and cleaning up food. Then there's emotional eating. Almost every adult has a childhood memory of food being used in a nurturing, rewarding, or punishing way. Food is one of the best "temporary" comforts we have. It is always there when we need it—when we are lonely, angry, disappointed, sad, or even happy. With hunger, malnutrition, anorexia, bulimia, compulsive eating, overeating, or just plain emotional eating, few people are exempt from having some kind of problem with food. And none of this is because of character weakness on our part. The food industry, our genetic make-up (we were designed to eat!), the media, and conflicting health and nutrition advice have all contributed to a society that spends a lot of money on food and subsequently on weight-loss—a futile cycle that endangers our health even more.

Let's face it—the health of our nation is poor. We have too much food at our fingertips and amazing technology that allows us to do virtually anything we want without moving a muscle. Over the past thirty years, the number of obese adults has increased 121 percent.[3,4]

But that's not the real tragedy. The number of overweight twelve- to nineteen-year-old children has increased 168 percent, and the number of overweight six- to eleven-year-olds has increased by a staggering 300 percent.[5,6] There are plenty of gloomy statistics one can recite to prove that our health is on the decline. But really, who wants to hear it? Just look around you. I sit at my desk day after day and email people who sit literally ten feet away from me—and not because I am lazy! I do this because I think I am too busy. We have all seen the evil workings of the adversary, but have we ever considered that maybe the adversary is waging a war on our health? Wouldn't it be easy for him to take away our health, happiness, and self-esteem in a technology-laden, food-dependent world? On the other hand, Heavenly Father wants us to be healthy; he gave us divine instruction pertaining to our temporal and spiritual health. As a beacon of light, he gave us the Word of Wisdom. The Word of Wisdom isn't just about what we *shouldn't* do but also about what we *should* do in order to *be our best.* For many of us, that means losing weight—and not just losing weight to fit into an item of clothing that was really bought too small as some sort of twisted motivation. Rather, it means losing weight to become healthy and feel great—so we can accomplish the great things Heavenly Father sent us here to do. The practical council of the "shoulds" of the Word of Wisdom will help us be physically healthy and spiritually strong. We all need to associate our personal health with the Word of Wisdom with a bit more zeal. In fact, doing so may just provide the motivation many of us need to achieve our health goals.

I am very proud to write this book in association with ICON Health & Fitness, one of the largest fitness companies in the world and a billion-dollar company. I am a registered dietitian, a certified personal trainer, and a manager for this amazing company. We see a nation in need of a solution—not another magic pill or potion, but a real solution for a real problem. Our purpose in writing this book is to spread the message of good health—nutritious meals, regular exercise, and a building up of the spirit. I must admit that I too enjoy eating delicious food (of course, that means chocolate) and succumbing to technological advances like my washing machine. It took me a while to acknowledge that as I was trying motivate others to "not use food as a comfort," and to have a hip-hip-hooray attitude about working out, I myself found food to be comforting and exercise a little inconvenient at times. However, through my experiences in this industry, I have learned what I have to do to account for my occasional unwise eating and exercise (or lack thereof) choices. I would like to share those tools with you.

This book covers the "Five Keys to Successful Weight Loss That Work." You may choose to work on one step at a time, or to put them all together for the maximum benefit: a life-changing, health-oriented approach to losing weight and feeling great. In the end, regardless of how many pounds you lose, your reward will be improved health. Moreover, as you read this book and implement the recommended lifestyle changes, I hope you experience some sort of epiphany—discovering the *real* benefit of healthy eating and regular exercise—vital, life-enhancing physical and spiritual health.

This book also includes quick and easy meal plans, delicious recipes, cardiovascular exercise programs, strength-training programs, tips for putting a program together that will work with *your* schedule, and how to move forward when you have had a bad day.

Within your grasp is a way of life that includes variety, balance, moderation, and sensibility—leading to weight loss, decreased risk or severity of disease, and improved overall health and well-being. Numerous research studies have shown that even simple lifestyle changes can lead to significant improvements in health. Empower yourself right now. Use the principles of the Word of Wisdom as your anchor. By doing so, you will find the strength to be your best. Not only do you deserve to be healthy, but when you're healthy, *life can be so much more.*

## The Word of Wisdom and Your Health

Heavenly Father created us, and only he knows what is best for our health. We need to be healthy so we can live happy, productive lives. We have families to protect, children to teach, and duties to the gospel. These precious human interactions are dependent on a healthy body, a healthy mind, and a healthy spirit.

There are both temporal and spiritual blessings that come from living the Word of Wisdom. All of us want to feel better, have more energy, and enjoy precious time with family and friends. The promise of the Word of Wisdom will bring us an increase of health, vitality, strength, endurance, greater resistance to disease, a savings of money not spent on wasteful food and harmful substances, and greater ability to resist temptation.[7]

The Lord gave the Word of Wisdom as a "principle with promise" (D&C 89:3). President Boyd K. Packer described a principle as the following: "A principle is an enduring truth, a law, a rule you can adopt to guide you in making decisions. Generally principles are not spelled out in detail. That leaves you free to find your way with an enduring truth, a principle, as your anchor."[8] Despite knowing this, many of us tend to want a detailed list of what is good and bad. Have you ever found yourself wondering, "Is white flour against the Word of Wisdom?" Or, "Is soda pop bad?" Joseph Fielding Smith stated, "Such revelation is unnecessary. The Word of Wisdom is a basic law. . . . Thus by keeping the commandment we are promised inspiration and the guidance of the Spirit of the Lord through which we will know what is good and what is bad for the body, without the Lord's presenting us with a detailed list separating the good things from the bad that we may be protected."[9] In other words, we need to apply the Word of Wisdom to our individual lifestyle habits as guided by the Spirit.

As part of my college education, I took classes in chemistry, biology, physiology, epidemiology, and, of course, nutrition. I am truly fascinated by the relevance of the Word of Wisdom in our society. Think about it: the Word of Wisdom was revealed in the year 1833. What did scientists know about nutrition at that time? What did they know about heart disease related to poor diet and inactivity? What did they know about tobacco and the risk of cancer? What did they know about the protective phytochemicals and antioxidants found in fruits and vegetables? The answer? Nothing. Almost two centuries old, the principles of the Word of Wisdom closely match the Dietary Guidelines for Americans 2005, which, based on the latest scientific evidence, state that fruit, vegetables, whole grains, low-fat milk products, lean meats, plant-based fats, and *prudence and moderation* promote good health and optimal well-being.

# The Do's of the Word of Wisdom

One of my favorite quotations about the Word of Wisdom simply states, "Those who are wise enough to practice the principle will reap its promised blessings."[10] Most of us are very familiar with the "should nots" of the Word of Wisdom. We know that alcohol, tobacco, and hot drinks are "not for the body" (D&C 89:8, 9). However, there is so much more to the Word of Wisdom. President Brigham Young said, "The blessings of food, sleep, and social enjoyment are ordained of God for his glory and our benefit, and it is for us to learn to use them and not abuse them, that his Kingdom may advance on the earth, and we advance in it."[11] In today's society, the abundance of food is a blessing that we have turned into a weakness by our own mismanagement. That's where the "do's" of the Word of Wisdom can help us be our best, physically and spiritually. Here is a review of what I think the Word of Wisdom tells us we "should" do:

## Wholesome Herbs to Be Used with Prudence

"All wholesome herbs God hath ordained for the constitution, nature, and use of man—every herb in the season thereof, and every fruit in the season thereof; all these to be used with prudence and thanksgiving" (D&C 89:10–11). The word herb refers to plants and vegetables that are nourishing and healthful for man. "In the season thereof" does not mean we can eat fruit and vegetables only at a certain time. Rather, these words mean that fresh foods have a superior value, and that we should not eat decaying or damaged foods. If fruits and vegetables are properly preserved, which is a common luxury in today's society, they should be enjoyed all through the year.[12] Why are we counseled to use these superior foods with "prudence and thanksgiving"? Use of the word *prudence* implies that good judgment—taking appropriate use and moderation into account—is needed. From a nutrition-science perspective, the answer is simple: Eating too much of anything is not healthy for the body. We should always practice moderation in all good things.

Nutritionally, fruits and vegetables are an amazing group of foods. They supply phyto-chemicals, a group of substances that plants naturally create as they try to protect them-selves against viruses and bacteria and seem to promote good health in humans. Current research has identified literally thousands of these protective phytochemicals that help pro-tect us from heart disease, some cancers, and other chronic health conditions.[13,14]

Fruits and vegetables are also high in fiber, low in calories, low in fat, and high in vita-mins and minerals. In addition, they are convenient, easy to prepare, and delicious. If the only change we made in our lives was to simply eat at least five servings (mind you, serving sizes are actually quite small) of fruits and vegetables each day, we could slash cancer rates by at least 20 percent.[15] The American Institute for Cancer Research has said that "there is a strong and consistent pattern showing that diets high in fruit and vegetables decrease the risk of many cancers, perhaps cancer in general." Specifically, diets high in fruits and veg-etables protect against cancers of the colon, stomach, rectum, esophagus, lungs, and phar-ynx. There is also sufficient evidence to suggest that diets high in fruits and vegetables probably protect against cancers of the breast, bladder, pancreas, and larynx.[16] Diets high in fruits and vegetables also protect against obesity and cardiovascular disease.[17] Despite all of this compelling research, more than 75 percent of Americans fail to meet the recommenda-tion of five servings per day.[18]

## Meat to Be Used Sparingly

"Yea, flesh also of beasts and of the fowls of the air, I, the Lord, have ordained for the use of man with thanksgiving; nevertheless they are to be used sparingly; and it is pleasing unto me that they should not be used, only in times of winter, or of cold, or famine" (D&C 89:12–13). With all of the fad diets that circulate in today's society, it is hard to not get caught up in extreme high-protein diets or total vegetarianism. The Word of Wisdom advocates neither. Consider another scripture, D&C 49:18–19: "Whoso forbiddeth to abstain from meats, that man should not eat the same, is not ordained of God; for, behold, the beasts of the field and the fowls of the air, and that which cometh of the earth, is ordained for the use of man for food and for raiment, and that he might have in abundance." The word *sparingly* refers to a "careful restraint" in respect to how often we eat meat, and how much of it we eat. For example, the recommended portion size of lean meat is three ounces—the approximate size and thickness of a deck of cards. Compare this small size to a gargantuan 64-ounce—yes, four-pound—slab of meat that we can order in some steakhouses. Now do you see the word "sparingly" in a different light?

The phrase "only in times of winter, or of cold, or famine" have caused many people to think that meat should be eaten only in the winter. However, when the Word of Wisdom was revealed, methods for preserving meat were primitive. We now know that storing meat at appropriate temperatures is vital to prevent serious and even fatal food-borne illnesses. Modern refrigeration now makes it easy for us to eat meat safely in any season. Overall, "the key word with respect to use of meat is 'sparingly.'"[19] However, remember that "sparingly" means different things to different people, depending on weight, age, and activity level. Apply the principles of the Word of Wisdom to your individual needs as guided by the Spirit.

Meat and meat products are a good source of many essential nutrients, including protein, iron, zinc, vitamin B12, and other vitamins and minerals. Meat also supplies us with fat (mainly saturated) and cholesterol—two food constituents the American diet is not deficient in. Current research tells us that a diet higher in red meat (beef, lamb, and pork) probably increases the risk for cancer of the colon and rectum, and possibly cancer of the breast, prostate, pancreas, and kidneys.[20] Additionally, the excess fat that comes from consuming too much meat puts us at risk for heart disease, some cancers, diabetes, and other health conditions associated with obesity. Many people eat meat for protein, protein, protein (we just can't get enough, right?). The truth is that the average American consumes adequate protein, and probably more than needed. Meat isn't our only source of protein. Protein is found in beans (or legumes), whole grains, vegetables, low-fat dairy products, eggs, cheese, nuts, and seeds.

## "All Grain Is Ordained for the Use of Man . . . to Be the Staff of Life"

"All grain is ordained for the use of man and of beasts, to be the staff of life, not only for man but for the beasts of the field, and the fowls of heaven, and all wild animals that run or creep on the earth" (D&C 89:14). "A staff is a support . . . that gives life to human beings."[21] The word "grain" refers to whole grains: wheat, brown rice, corn, oatmeal, whole-grain cereals, and whole wheat breads. One problem with the current food guide pyramid is that most Americans relate the guideline of "6–11 servings daily of bread, cereal, rice and pasta" to the commonly served refined breads, rice, pasta, and sugary cereals. I am sure the Lord did not intend for us to eat 1,000-calorie cinnamon rolls, platters of pasta, and single muffins that serve four as the "staff of life."

Whole grains are low in fat and cholesterol and rich in "healthy" carbohydrates, fiber, vitamins, minerals, and phytochemicals. These foods are also excellent sources of thiamin (B1), riboflavin (B2), niacin (B3), vitamin B6, folic acid, and other vitamins and trace minerals. With such a diverse offering of nutrition and a wide variety of options, it is easy to see why the Lord revealed grains to be the "staff of life."

President Ezra Taft Benson summed up wholesome living and the Word of Wisdom in one amazing quotation: "The condition of the physical body can affect the spirit. That's why the Lord gave us the Word of Wisdom. He also said that we should retire to our beds early and arise early (see D&C 88:124), that we should not run faster than we have strength (see D&C 10:4), and that we should use moderation in all good things. . . . Food can affect the mind, and deficiencies in certain elements in the body can promote mental depression. . . . Rest and physical exercise are essential, and a walk in the fresh air can refresh the spirit. Wholesome recreation is part of our religion, and a change of pace is necessary, and even its anticipation can lift the spirit."[22]

## Putting the Word of Wisdom into Practice

Putting knowledge into practice is always difficult. Even though the health recommendations from the Word of Wisdom and current scientific research seem basic enough, the current state of health in this nation speaks for itself. The U.S. Department of Health and Human Services and the U.S. Department of Agriculture have said that "Americans must make significant changes in their eating habits and lifestyles" to correct the problem of overweight, obesity, and chronic disease.[23] "Significant changes" doesn't mean memorizing the calorie content of the thousands of foods on the market. And it certainly doesn't mean exercising to the point of collapse. Rather, we just need to *follow through* with the basic principles of good nutrition and daily exercise. All of our good intentions—whether it be to eat whole-wheat bread instead of white or to give up that morning Snickers and Coke—have to become actions. These kinds of small daily achievements really can add up to big changes in our health. Granted, losing weight and eating well is not that black-and-white. Questions pertaining to portion size, food labeling and manufacturing, the uncertain calorie content of home-prepared meals, restaurant meals, and unlabeled foods along with questions pertaining to the how, when, where, and what of exercise all contribute to the tendency to stick to our old ways. That's why the rest of this book is devoted to helping you:

1. Increase your knowledge of nutrition and exercise so that you can make informed decisions about your health.

2. Learn easy tips and guidelines that will help you overcome barriers to eating right and exercising regularly.

3. Learn simple ways to implement balance, variety, and moderation-based habits into your lifestyle.

This book can and will help you put your weight-loss and good-health intentions into practice. I have summarized the latest research on nutrition, exercise, weight management, and the teachings of the Word of Wisdom into "Five Keys to Successful Weight Loss That Work." Remember, if it helps you stick with the program, pick one step to work on at a time. However, for maximum benefit, use all five steps together on an average daily basis. These steps were designed to be simple and easy to understand and to help you become a leaner, healthier person. They were also designed to be implementable and maintainable—*for a lifetime.*

## Notes

1. J. Kruger, D. A. Galuska, M. K. Serdula, and D. A. Jones, "Attempting to Lose Weight: Specific Practices among U.S. Adults," *American Journal of Preventative Medicine,* June 2004; 26(5):402–6.

2. A. A. Hedley, C. L. Ogden, C. L. Johnson, M. D. Carroll, L. R. Curtin, and K. M. Flegal, "Prevalence of Overweight and Obesity among U.S. Children, Adolescents, and Adults, 1999–2002," *Journal of the American Medical Association,* 2004; 291(23):2847–50.

3. A. A. Hedley, C. L. Ogden, C. L. Johnson, M. D. Carroll, L. R. Curtin, and K. M. Flegal, "Prevalence of Overweight and Obesity among U.S. Children, Adolescents, and Adults, 1999–2002," *Journal of the American Medical Association,* 2004; 291(23):2847–50.

4. *Chartbook on Trends in Health of Americans 2003* (Centers for Disease Control and Prevention, National Center for Health Statistics, National Health Examination Survey and National Health and Nutrition Survey).

5. A. A. Hedley, C. L. Ogden, C. L. Johnson, M. D. Carroll, L. R. Curtin, and K. M. Flegal, "Prevalence of Overweight and Obesity among U.S. Children, Adolescents, and Adults, 1999–2002," *Journal of the American Medical Association*, 2004; 291(23):2847–50.

6. *Chartbook on Trends in Health of Americans 2003* (Centers for Disease Control and Prevention, National Center for Health Statistics, National Health Examination Survey and National Health and Nutrition Survey).

7. *Doctrine and Covenants Student Manual* (Salt Lake City: The Church of Jesus Christ of Latter-day Saints, 1981), 206–11.

8. Boyd K. Packer, "The Word of Wisdom: The Principle and the Promises," *Ensign*, May 1996, 17.

9. *Improvement Era*, February 1956, 78–79.

10. Stephen E. Robinson and H. Dean Garrett, *A Commentary on the Doctrine and Covenants*, 4 vols. (Salt Lake City: Deseret Book, 2004), 3:144–45.

11. *Journal of Discourses*, 26 vols. (London: Latter-day Saints' Book Depot, 1854–86), 6:149.

12. *Doctrine and Covenants Student Manual* (Salt Lake City: The Church of Jesus Christ of Latter-day Saints, 1981), 209.

13. Roberta L. Duyff, *The American Dietetic Association's Complete Food and Nutrition Guide* (Chronimed Publishing, 1998), 149.

14. *Simple Steps to Prevent Cancer* [brochure] (Washington, D.C.: American Institute for Cancer Research, 2000).

15. *Simple Steps to Prevent Cancer* [brochure] (Washington, D.C.: American Institute for Cancer Research, 2000).

16. Geoffrey Cannon, ed., *Food, Nutrition, and the Prevention of Cancer: A Global Perspective* (New York: American Institute for Cancer Research and BANTA Book Group, 1997), 515.

17. Geoffrey Cannon, ed., *Food, Nutrition, and the Prevention of Cancer: A Global Perspective* (New York: American Institute for Cancer Research and BANTA Book Group, 1997), 440.

18. *Behavioral Risk Factor Surveillance Survey* (Nationwide 2003 Prevalence Data), http://apps.nccd.cdc.gov/brfss/display.asp?cat=FV&yr=2003&qkey=4415&state=US.

19. *Doctrine and Covenants Student Manual* (Salt Lake City: The Church of Jesus Christ of Latter-day Saints, 1981), 210.

20. Geoffrey Cannon, ed., *Food, Nutrition, and the Prevention of Cancer: A Global Perspective* (New York: American Institute for Cancer Research and BANTA Book Group, 1997), 515.

21. Stephen E. Robinson and H. Dean Garrett, *A Commentary on the Doctrine and Covenants*, 4 vols. (Salt Lake City: Deseret Book, 2004), 3:150.

22. Ezra Taft Benson, in *Peace* (Salt Lake City: Deseret Book, 1998), 37.

23. *Dietary Guidelines for Americans 2005* (Washington, D.C.: U.S. Department of Health and Human Services and the U.S. Department of Agriculture).

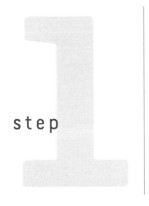

# Think Healthy, Not Skinny

**KEY POINTS:**
Discovering the True Meaning of Good Health | Understanding Disease Risk and Your Health Status | Building a Positive Body Image in a Negative World | Connecting Your Mind, Body, and Spirit | Learning to Forget "Diets" | Understanding Metabolism

## The True Meaning of Good Health

Focusing on health is important because the state of our health can affect every aspect of our lives—our work, our play, our social behavior, our daily interactions with family members, and even our faithfulness to the Church. Take a few moments to think about what good health means to you. Does it have a certain look? I hope not. Good health is not defined by a dress size, a waistline, or a bustline; good health is a lifestyle. "For the health professional, health is defined as an independent, nondieting lifestyle characterized by nourishing eating and activity patterns, and self-acceptance."[1] To apply that meaning in real life, it means putting aside the scale, listening to your body, eating when your body says "more" and stopping when your body says "enough," discovering your own food and activity patterns to keep you energized, and most important, finding the inner strength to accept yourself just as you are and move on with life.[2] We now know that exercise is a powerful promoter of health and longevity regardless of what the number is on the bathroom scale. Many studies have shown an "unequivocal and robust relation of fitness, physical activity, and exercise" to lower death rates and reduce cardiovascular risk.[3] A compelling study done by the Cooper Institute of Health found that lean, unfit men had double the risk of all-cause mortality compared to lean, fit mean. A low fitness level was also associated with a higher risk for cardiovascular disease mortality.[4] Just because someone is a size 6 doesn't mean that her heart is strong, her cholesterol is low, and her blood pressure is stable. Likewise, just because someone is heavy doesn't mean that she is lazy, sedentary, and unfit. In fact, in 1997 the American Institute for Cancer Research issued a landmark research report in which scientists estimated that the incidence of cancer could be reduced by a staggering 30 to 40 percent simply by eating a healthy diet, getting regular physical activity, and maintaining a healthy weight. This report remains the most comprehensive ever done (it analyzed more than 4,500 studies) regarding cancer and diet.[5] The bottom line is that, regardless of body size, regular physical activity and basic healthful nutrition habits are essential for good health.

## Disease Risk and Your Health Status

So yes, just because you are skinny doesn't mean you are off the "must-get-healthy" hook. But excess pounds do raise your risk for certain diseases. Hardly a day goes by without someone you know being affected in some way by heart disease, adult-onset diabetes, high blood pressure, arthritis, or cancer. All of these diseases are associated with excess weight. Harvard's Walter Willet says "avoiding weight gain, along with not smoking, is one of the most important things people can do to protect their long term health."[6] The research goes on and on; even the centers for Disease Control has stated that the obesity epidemic has devastating impacts on health, quality of life, and health care costs.[7] If we know that excess pounds are killing us, then we know that excess pounds are not good for our health. Period. We do know that the location of the excess fat plays a role in disease risk. Fat tissue in the abdominal and chest area (also known as an "apple" shape) seems to be much more detrimental to health than fat tissue around the hips and thighs (also known as a "pear" shape). The good news is that, for some diseases, the weight loss doesn't have to be huge. In one Harvard study, women who reported losing only about ten pounds lowered their risk of diabetes by 80 percent.[8]

So that brings me back to my lifelong motto: "Everything you do counts." Even small attempts to improve your health will provide some benefit. Even if you are at risk for or already suffer from heart disease, adult-onset diabetes, high blood pressure, or cancer— eating healthfully and engaging in regular physical activity can reduce your risk for the disease, improve your condition, and in some cases even *reverse* your condition. You have to start somewhere. If you can at least get on the right path, you will achieve better health in the long run.

## Building a Positive Body Image in a Negative World

Besides taking care of our bodies, we need to improve our minds. The first time I watched a graphic designer use a computer mouse to alter a photograph and "shave" off the hips of a young model, I was horrified. That was just the beginning; I then learned that most models on the covers of magazines have been airbrushed, blended, smoothed, brightened, and fixed in just the right areas. That was it—I decided my overwhelming feelings of inadequacy every time I walked past a magazine with a "perfect" model on the cover were ludicrous. Why compare ourselves to something seemingly perfect, when we all know that every person in this world is imperfect? Don't let marketers and the media tell you that you're the wrong shape, or that you have to starve, alter, or manipulate your body to fit a fad. One of my favorite quotations simply states, "There are three billion women who don't look like supermodels, and only eight who do" (The Body Shop). How many times have we all said to ourselves, "If I can just lose a few pounds then I will be happier?" The truth is that body image and weight loss are two different things. Even when diets help us lose a few pounds, there is always something more—"I should lose *just a few* more pounds"; "I need to get rid of the flab under my arms"; "I still have too many wrinkles"—that gets in the way of allowing ourselves to have a positive body image. The truth is, no matter what your size, you need to accept yourself, right now, for who you are. Sound difficult? Why don't you try this exercise to help you explore all the amazing things about yourself that you really should learn to appreciate:

First, grab a sheet of paper and draw your best impression of a human silhouette (this is the hardest part for me; drawing is not even in my scope of potential talents). Draw the fingers, toes, eyes, ears, nose, and mouth. Go for it; make this something you can be proud of.

Second, sit back and think about your qualities. Are you a good listener? Do you play the piano? Do you crochet beautiful things that bring warmth on cold days? Maybe you see good where others see bad. Do you have a warm heart? Are you quick to remember dates, names, and times?

Third, write down each quality next to the correlating body part. A warm heart goes on the chest. Playing beautiful music goes on the fingers. And so on.

Finally, put the picture where you will see it often: in your journal, on your fridge, or maybe on the inside of your closet.

This exercise will help you focus on liking yourself for who you are on the inside—not on the outside. If you can learn to love yourself in any size or shape, you will have a positive self-image in a negative world.

## Connecting Mind, Body, and Spirit

Connecting your mind, body, and spirit means having a healthy body image, a healthy body, and a strong spirit. Elder Russell M. Nelson said this: "Remarkable as your body is, its prime purpose is of even greater importance—to serve as tenement for your spirit. . . . Not an age in life passes without temptation, trial, or torment experienced through your physical body. But as you prayerfully develop self-mastery, desires of the flesh may be subdued. And when that has been achieved, you may have the strength to submit to your Heavenly Father, as did Jesus, who said, 'Not my will, but thine, be done.'" (Luke 22:42.) . . . Physical conditioning through regular exercise requires self-mastery too. I marvel at Elder Joseph Anderson, now in his ninety-sixth year. For decades, the strength of his spirit over his body has induced him to swim regularly. But his motivation has never been to attain physical longevity; that has come only incidentally. His desire has been to serve God and His anointed. Elder Anderson has followed what I label as the Lord's prescription for a long and useful life. Those faithful in 'magnifying their calling, are sanctified by the Spirit unto the renewing of their bodies. They become . . . the elect of God.' (D&C 84:33–34.)"[9] There are several scriptures that specifically address our health and the important connection between our mind, body, and spirit.

1. "The spirit and the body are the soul of man." (D&C 88:15.)

2. "All things unto me are spiritual, and not at any time have I given unto you a law which was temporal; neither any man, nor the children of men; neither Adam, your father, whom I created. Behold, I gave unto him that he should be an agent unto himself; and I gave unto him commandment, but no temporal commandment gave I unto him, for my commandments are spiritual; they are not natural nor temporal, neither carnal nor sensual." (D&C 29:34–35.) (Application: All commandments are spiritual; things that hurt the body also hurt the spirit.)

3. "Cease to be idle; cease to be unclean; cease to find fault one with another; cease to sleep longer than is needful; retire to thy bed early, that ye may not be weary; arise early, that your bodies and your minds may be invigorated." (D&C 88:124.) (Application: These are general rules of physical and spiritual health.[10])

4. "All saints who remember to keep and do these sayings, walking in obedience to the commandments, shall receive health in their navel and marrow to their

bones." (D&C 89:18.) (Application: "Promised blessings of physical health are but the means to greater spiritual achievement."[11])

The scriptures are full of gospel teachings promoting our temporal and spiritual growth and development. Always remember how vital, yet fragile, that connection between your mind, body, and spirit really is.

## Forget "Diets"

**di·et**

*Etymology: Middle English diete, from Old French, from Latin diaeta, from Greek diaita, literally, manner of living, from diaitasthai to lead one's life 1 a : food and drink regularly provided or consumed. b : habitual nourishment. c : the kind and amount of food prescribed for a person or animal for a special reason.*

*Deprivation. Restriction. Poor self-control. Guilt. Punishment.* These words were never intended to define the word *diet.* Over the years, the word has been molded and shaped to fit the needs of a culture obsessed with appearance. Diets, as we view them today, can have many negative effects on our lives. I have never before felt the urge to search through the sea of diet-related internet claims. However, late one summer evening, as I stared blankly at my computer, I took the plunge and typed in the word *diet* for an internet search. Amazingly, it took a mere one-tenth of a second to generate a list exceeding more than 27,500,000 results. Wow! I then tried to narrow my search to just books; I typed in the word *diet* on Amazon.com and within seconds had more than 105,356 different books from which to choose. Clearly, there are too many fad diets out there. The rule of thumb is that "if it sounds too good to be true, it probably is." Diets that tell you a specific food group is toxic to your body (those poor carbohydrates!) are, on the average, ill-advised. Think about the vast diversity of diets that human beings have survived on for thousands of years—and continue to survive on in our current day. We have cultures that survive on high-carbohydrate diets (African and Asian countries), cultures that enjoy diets higher in monounsaturated fats (like the Mediterranean diet from Southern Europe),[12] and cultures that continually overindulge in meat and fat. All cultures eat differently, yet we all survive. We may not be our healthiest, but we all survive.

Aside from the negative metabolic and emotional consequences, diets can quickly sever the delicate balance of a healthy mind, body, and spirit. Besides that, diets wreak havoc on our metabolism.

## Understanding Metabolism

Let's start with the basics. The human body was designed to do exactly what was needed for thousands of years—survive when food was scarce. It wasn't until the past twenty or thirty years that we began to have enormously abundant and readily accessible sources of food. Your body needs calories to maintain precious body tissue. Preserving muscle tissue requires more calories than preserving fat tissue. (Fat tissue requires only a few meager calories to function, yet fat tissue appears to be active in secreting or stimulating hormones that affect our health.) So when you drastically cut your calorie intake, your body begins to search for ways to distribute calories wisely to preserve vital organs and tissues. Muscle is one of the first things to go. Fat is also lost, but at the same time your body preferentially stores fat tissue, saving it for a later time if the food scarcity continues. The cycle doesn't end there, even when calorie intake returns to normal. Your body can't just forget that stark experience, and it continues to store fat in case of another food shortage. In addition, the basal metabolism—the amount of calories your body burns at rest to feed muscles, tissues, and organs—is now lower because of the loss of natural calorie-burning muscle tissue. This whole process is powerful and complicated yet almost foolproof as your complex metabolic circuitry tightly regulates your body weight, energy intake, and energy expenditure.[13]

Here's an example of what I mean:

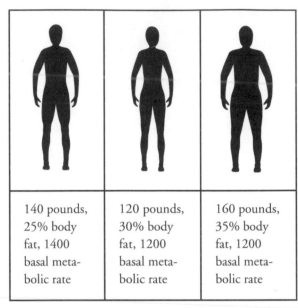

| 140 pounds, 25% body fat, 1400 basal metabolic rate | 120 pounds, 30% body fat, 1200 basal metabolic rate | 160 pounds, 35% body fat, 1200 basal metabolic rate |

*[Illustration 1–1]*

Sue started out at 140 pounds, 25 percent body fat, and a metabolic rate of 1,400 (the number of calories her body uses to feed muscles, tissues, and organs at rest). She goes on a crash diet, eating only 900 calories per day with no exercise. She loses 20 pounds (see illustration 1-1), 10 pounds of muscle and 10 pounds of fat. She is now at 21 percent body fat, and her metabolic rate has dropped by 200 calories per day, to only 1,200. After completing the six-week crash diet, she goes back to eating her previous high-calorie diet. Because her metabolism is now slower, needing 200 calories less per day, her body begins to store the now-extra calories as fat. The result? Three months later she ends up with ten extra pounds, 35 percent body fat, and a sluggish metabolism—essentially worse off metabolically than when she started.

So now we know why dieting is so hard on our metabolism, but here's the million-dollar question: How do we *raise* our metabolism? The answer? Eating and exercising. First, eating small (think small!) amounts of food more often throughout the day stimulates a healthy, active metabolism. Compare this to skipping breakfast, skipping lunch, and then eating a monstrous dinner. In this scenario, your metabolism is practically dormant all day and then suddenly has a good 1,000 to 2,000 calories to deal with all at once (perfect timing, as the next step is to go to bed and burn very few calories all night). The second way we can boost our metabolism is through regular exercise. This is the only way to build lean muscle (not big, bulky muscles but lean, healthy muscle tissue), and adding muscle means our body needs more calories at rest, and even during exercise, to function. Hence, an increase in metabolic rate.

Calories are important. You need to eat enough calories every day to at least meet your resting energy needs. You need to stay active to keep your muscle tissue strong and active. You don't have to calorie-count to be healthy; you just need to use moderation and listen to your body's internal cues that tell you to eat when you are hungry and stop when you are full. The word *full* doesn't mean to eat until you are sick and uncomfortable; it simply means eating until you are *no longer hungry*. Big difference. Here is a chart that explains why and how your body uses calories:

| % DAILY CALORIE NEEDS | PURPOSE | FUNCTIONS | AFFECTED BY "DIETING"? |
|---|---|---|---|
| 60% | Basal Metabolic Rate | The energy used for your heart to beat, your lungs to breathe, your muscles to move, your hair to grow, your skin, and all other bodily functions | Yes, losing weight without exercising merely by eating too few calories results in a loss of metabolically active muscle tissue and therefore lowers metabolic rate |
| 30% | Physical Activity | Includes everything from getting out of bed to ultra-high-intensity workouts | Yes, losing muscle means less calories are burned during physical activity |
| 10% | Digestion and Absorption of Food | Energy required to break down and properly use the food you eat | Yes, eating less means you expend less energy to digest food |

[*Illustration 1–2*]

For the 65 percent of us that are classified as overweight by the government, we do need to cut back on calories, but we don't need to go on a very low-calorie diet. Even though I have spent many pages telling you that good health is not tied to a specific number on the bathroom scale, it is important to realize that if you are not exercising regularly and eating healthfully then you need to take the necessary steps to improve your health and possibly lose a few pounds. I am not going to tell you what you should or shouldn't weigh, because I think most of us just *know* when we are not at our best. The chart below will help you assess your weight by comparing yourself to current government standards.

## Weight Chart

Directions: 1. Look on the left and find your height. 2. Go across to the right and find your weight. 3. Now go up and see if your weight is a "Good Weight" or a weight with "Increasing Risk" associated with it. If you found that you have an increased risk assigned to your weight, then it is highly recommended that you lose 10% or more of your current weight to reduce your risk factors.

### Table of Body Mass Index (BMI)*

| Your BMI | 19 | 20 | 21 | 22 | 23 | 24 | 25 | 26 | 27 | 28 | 29 | 30 | 31 | 32 | 33 | 34 | 35 | 36 | 37 | 38 | 39 | 40 |
|---|---|---|---|---|---|---|---|---|---|---|---|---|---|---|---|---|---|---|---|---|---|---|
| Your Height | GOOD WEIGHTS | | | | | | | <INCREASING RISKS> | | | | | | | | | | | | | | |
| 4'10" | 91 | 96 | 100 | 105 | 110 | 115 | 119 | 124 | 129 | 134 | 138 | 143 | 148 | 153 | 158 | 162 | 167 | 172 | 177 | 181 | 186 | 191 |
| 4'11" | 94 | 99 | 104 | 109 | 114 | 119 | 124 | 128 | 133 | 138 | 143 | 148 | 153 | 158 | 163 | 168 | 173 | 178 | 183 | 188 | 193 | 198 |
| 5' | 97 | 102 | 107 | 112 | 118 | 123 | 128 | 133 | 138 | 143 | 148 | 153 | 158 | 163 | 168 | 174 | 179 | 184 | 189 | 194 | 199 | 204 |
| 5'1" | 100 | 106 | 111 | 116 | 122 | 127 | 132 | 137 | 143 | 148 | 153 | 158 | 164 | 169 | 174 | 180 | 185 | 190 | 195 | 201 | 206 | 211 |
| 5'2" | 104 | 109 | 115 | 120 | 126 | 131 | 136 | 142 | 147 | 153 | 158 | 164 | 169 | 175 | 180 | 186 | 191 | 196 | 202 | 207 | 213 | 218 |
| 5'3" | 107 | 113 | 118 | 124 | 130 | 135 | 141 | 146 | 152 | 158 | 163 | 169 | 175 | 180 | 186 | 191 | 197 | 203 | 208 | 214 | 220 | 225 |
| 5'4" | 110 | 116 | 122 | 128 | 134 | 140 | 145 | 151 | 157 | 163 | 169 | 174 | 180 | 186 | 192 | 197 | 204 | 209 | 215 | 221 | 227 | 232 |
| 5'5" | 114 | 120 | 126 | 132 | 138 | 144 | 150 | 156 | 162 | 168 | 174 | 180 | 186 | 192 | 198 | 204 | 210 | 216 | 222 | 228 | 234 | 240 |
| 5'6" | 118 | 124 | 130 | 136 | 142 | 148 | 155 | 161 | 167 | 173 | 179 | 186 | 192 | 198 | 204 | 210 | 216 | 223 | 229 | 235 | 241 | 247 |
| 5'7" | 121 | 127 | 134 | 140 | 146 | 153 | 159 | 166 | 172 | 178 | 185 | 191 | 198 | 204 | 211 | 217 | 223 | 230 | 236 | 242 | 249 | 255 |
| 5'8" | 125 | 131 | 138 | 144 | 151 | 158 | 164 | 171 | 177 | 184 | 190 | 197 | 203 | 210 | 216 | 223 | 230 | 236 | 243 | 249 | 256 | 262 |
| 5'9" | 128 | 135 | 142 | 149 | 155 | 162 | 169 | 176 | 182 | 189 | 196 | 203 | 209 | 216 | 223 | 230 | 236 | 243 | 250 | 257 | 263 | 270 |
| 5'10" | 132 | 139 | 146 | 153 | 160 | 167 | 174 | 181 | 188 | 195 | 202 | 209 | 216 | 222 | 229 | 236 | 243 | 250 | 257 | 264 | 271 | 278 |
| 5'11" | 136 | 143 | 150 | 157 | 165 | 172 | 179 | 186 | 193 | 200 | 208 | 215 | 222 | 229 | 236 | 243 | 250 | 257 | 265 | 272 | 279 | 286 |
| 6' | 140 | 147 | 154 | 162 | 169 | 177 | 184 | 191 | 199 | 206 | 213 | 221 | 228 | 235 | 242 | 250 | 258 | 265 | 272 | 279 | 287 | 294 |
| 6'1" | 144 | 151 | 159 | 166 | 174 | 182 | 189 | 197 | 204 | 212 | 219 | 227 | 235 | 242 | 250 | 257 | 265 | 272 | 280 | 288 | 295 | 302 |
| 6'2" | 148 | 155 | 163 | 171 | 179 | 186 | 194 | 202 | 210 | 218 | 225 | 233 | 241 | 249 | 256 | 264 | 272 | 280 | 287 | 295 | 303 | 311 |
| 6'3" | 152 | 160 | 168 | 176 | 184 | 192 | 200 | 208 | 216 | 224 | 232 | 240 | 248 | 256 | 264 | 272 | 279 | 287 | 295 | 303 | 311 | 319 |
| 6'4" | 156 | 164 | 172 | 180 | 189 | 197 | 205 | 213 | 221 | 230 | 238 | 246 | 254 | 263 | 271 | 279 | 287 | 295 | 304 | 312 | 320 | 328 |

*[Illustration 1–3]*

*Please note that BMI calculations are just one indication of healthy body weight, and there are individual differences. Those who have very low body fat (i.e. athletes), age less than 19 years of age or 70+, pregnant/breastfeeding women, or the chronically ill, may require other indicators. Source: George A. Bray, Contemporary Diagnosis and Management of Obesity, Handbooks in Health Care, 1998.*

The traditional rule is that if you want to lose one pound per week, you should create a calorie deficiency of 3,500 calories per week. This can be done through extra exercise or by cutting 500 calories per day from your food intake. My preference for any good weight-management program is a cut of 300 to 500 calories per day and at least thirty minutes of exercise on most days of the week. This combination often results in a loss of one to two pounds per week, which is safe, realistic, and most important, maintainable. For most people who are overweight, a decrease of 500 calories per day will not push the body into crisis survival mode. Healthful weight management programs that recommend a realistic cut in calories, include all food groups in moderation, and promote regular physical activity are the best programs for weight loss, improved health, and decreased risk of disease.

So yes, forget the "Sure-Fire, Lightning-Fast, Hunger-Free, Easy-As-Pie, Just-4-You, Permanent-Weight-Loss, Health-and-Happiness Diet"[14]—or any other diet that makes similar claims. From here on out, diet means "food for habitual nourishment" and "manner of living." And remember, diet is about how you live, not how you don't. Focus on health, not weight. Set a goal to exercise or eat right because you want to be healthy, not so you can see a specific number on your bathroom scale.

## Notes

1. Kathy King Helm and Bridget Klawitter, "Nutrition Therapy Advanced Counseling Skills" (adapted and reprinted with permission of Linda Omihinski, *Healthy Weight Journal,* vol. 9, no. 1; 1995).

2. Kathy King Helm and Bridget Klawitter, "Nutrition Therapy Advanced Counseling Skills" (adapted and reprinted with permission of Linda Omihinski, *Healthy Weight Journal,* vol. 9, no. 1; 1995).

3. C. D. Lee, S. N. Blair, and A. S. Jackson, "Cardiorespiratory Fitness, Body Composition, and All-Cause and Cardiovascular Disease Mortality in Men," *American Journal of Clinical Nutrition,* 1999; 69(3):373–380.

4. G. J. Balady, "Survival of the Fittest—More Evidence," *New England Journal of Medicine,* 2002; 346(11):852.

5. Geoffrey Cannon, ed., *Food, Nutrition, and the Prevention of Cancer: A Global Perspective* (New York: American Institute for Cancer Research and BANTA Book Group, 1997), 7.

6. Bonnie Liebman, *Nutrition Action,* vol. 9 no. 8, October 2003 (Center for Science in the Public Interest).

7. www.cdc.gov/PDF/Frequently_asked_questions_about_calculating_Obesity-related_risk.pdf.

8. Bonnie Liebman, Nutrition Action, vol. 9 no. 8, October 2003 (Center for Science in the Public Interest).

9. Russell M. Nelson, "Self-Mastery," *Ensign,* November 1985, 30.

10. *Doctrine and Covenants Student Manual* (Salt Lake City: The Church of Jesus Christ of Latter-day Saints, 1981), 206–11.

11. *Doctrine and Covenants Student Manual* (Salt Lake City: The Church of Jesus Christ of Latter-day Saints, 1981), 206–11.

12. Geoffrey Cannon, ed., *Food, Nutrition, and the Prevention of Cancer: A Global Perspective* (New York: American Institute for Cancer Research and BANTA Book Group, 1997), 24.

13. J. Korner, R. L. Leibel, "To Eat or Not to Eat—How the Gut Talks to the Brain," *New England Journal of Medicine,* 2003; 349:926–28.

14. Bonnie Liebman, Nutrition Action, vol. 31, no. 1, January/February 2004 (Center for Science in the public Interest).

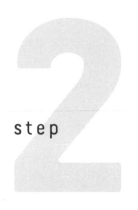

# Eat Sensibly

**KEY POINTS:**
Understanding the Food Industry and Our Culture | Learning to Read the Nutrition Label | Understanding Portion Control | Healthy Eating Guidelines: Plant-based foods—Healthy fats—Lean meats and other protein-rich foods—Calcium—Tips for eating on the run | A Summary for Eating Sensibly

step

## The Food Industry and Our Culture

If you think you are in the midst of a food fight, you are not alone. Dave Barry, who never fails to make me laugh, wrote a funny article on this very topic. "One recent Tuesday morning," he wrote, "I was flipping through the TV channels at a brisk, businesslike, no-nonsense pace, looking for 'Rocky and Bullwinkle,' when I found myself caught up in a fascinating installment of Leeza Gibbons' talk show, 'Leeza.' The theme of the show was: . . . 'Superstars of the Diet Wars.' This was a debate among top diet experts who felt so strongly about the correct way to lose weight that at times they came close to whacking each other over the head with their competing diet books. Dieting was not always so complicated. Thousands of years ago, there was only one diet book, entitled 'Don't Eat Too Much.' It consisted of a big stone tablet on which were chiseled the words 'DON'T EAT TOO MUCH!' It did not sell well, because nobody could lift it, on top of which everybody back then was busy with other concerns, such as not starving. In modern America, however, food is abundant everywhere except aboard commercial airplanes. Dieting has become a huge industry involving many complex theories that can be confusing to the average layperson sitting on the Barcalounger, trying to decide whether to open a second bag of potato chips or simply eat the onion dip right out of the tub."[1]

Hardly a day goes by without the media reporting more staggering statistics about the poor health of our nation and who is to blame for it. Some believe the food industry is to blame. Some believe the problem is genetic. Some believe the problem is a result of our own actions. And some believe it comes from our sedentary environment and a never-ending food supply. I believe our health problems are a result of all these things. We have the ability to change our actions and our sedentary lifestyles. However, we don't have the ability to change our genes. And at this point, we certainly don't have the ability to control the way the food industry spends billions of dollars every year to continually spit out ads for sugary sodas, cereals, snack foods, junk foods, and high-fat foods. The result: a relentless pressure to eat unhealthy foods. Think about it. When was the last time you saw an ad for scrumptious strawberries? Crunchy carrots? The answer? Likely never.

Food is available everywhere: convenience stores, shopping malls, airports, sporting events, grocery stores, movie theaters, schools, and practically every corner. The U.S. food supply provides us with 3,900 calories per day—that's almost double the amount most of us need.[2] In his usual up-front manner, Brigham Young once said, "The Americans, as a nation, are killing themselves with their vices and high living. As much as a man ought to eat in half an hour they swallow in three minutes, gulping down their food like the [dog] under the table, which, when a chunk of meat is thrown down to it, swallows it before you can say 'twice.' If you want a reform, carry out the advice I have just given you. Dispense with your multitudinous dishes, and, depend upon it, you will do much towards preserving your families from sickness, disease, and death."[3] Now, Brigham Young said this sometime in the mid-1850s. What do you think he would say about our ability to gulp down excess amounts of food in today's times? I can think of many times when I have "gulped down" a large portion of food—in *less* than three minutes! Even though we have many choices in relation to food and drink, we know that the Lord expects us to use our own wise judgment when it comes to making all life choices, including those related to our health. In D&C 58:27–28 he says, "Men should be anxiously engaged in a good cause, and do many things of their own free will. . . . For the power is in them, wherein they are agents unto themselves."

We live in a world where we can access a host of nutrition advice—some helpful, some shady, and some outright dangerous. Of course, the internet is a major link between the average consumer and nutrition information. But even cereal boxes and cans of soup are touting "clinical studies" showing that these products these products fight a certain disease or ailment. Before trying to search for accurate nutrition advice on your own, seek out a registered dietitian, food scientist, or medical doctor. A "nutritionist" doesn't necessarily have a degree, and there are no governing agencies regulating qualifications for people who call themselves nutritionists. In reviewing "clinical studies," look for those that have been published in a credible "peer-reviewed" journal such as the *Journal of the American Medical Association* or the *New England Journal of Medicine*.

## Reading the Nutrition Label

In 1973 the U.S. Food and Drug Administration established a system to provide select nutrition information for certain foods. In 1990 food labels were revised and updated through the Nutrition Labeling and Education Act. At present, the U.S. Food and Drug Administration has the authority to require and regulate nutrition labeling for most foods, while the U.S. Department of Agriculture regulates meat and poultry products. The nutrition label includes a lot of useful information that, if you take a moment to review it, could help you make drastic changes in your health.

This is the label for a 20-ounce bottle of soda pop. How many calories does this bottle contain? If you said 100, you just fell victim to a common misinterpretation of food labels. This product actually has 250 calories for the entire 20-ounce bottle—which is what most people consume. This is not unique; you will see the same thing on many food products. Here's a review of what is on a label, why you need to know about it, and how you can interpret the information correctly.

## Nutrition Facts

Serving Size 8 fl oz (240 mL)
Servings Per Container 2.5

**Amount Per Serving**

Calories 100

| | % Daily Value* |
|---|---|
| Total Fat 0g | 0% |
| Sodium 30mg | 1% |
| Total Carbohydrate 31g | 10% |
| Sugars 31g | |
| Protein 0g | |

*Not a significant source of other nutrients.*

*Percent Daily Values are based on a 2,000 calorie diet.

*Serving Size and Servings Per Container.* This information is crucial. If you don't read anything else on the label, at least look at how many servings are in the container so you don't gobble up four servings unknowingly. All of the information (calories, fat, sodium, cholesterol, fiber—everything except the food ingredients) is based on the specified serving size. Serving size is not based on the amount you actually *eat*. Serving size is standardized by the government and based on how much of the food people *usually* eat—and although serving sizes are consistent among similar products, in some instances they seem to be on the small side in comparison to the amount of food we eat in real life. Yes, we should drink only 8 ounces of soda at one sitting, but how many of us actually save the other 60 percent of the beverage for another time? Although government regulations are extremely helpful, we as consumers don't seem to fully comprehend the information on the food label. The government has standardized the portion size, not the container size; but consumers are under the illusion that the portion size is often the container size. Here's another example of what I mean.

This label is for a cookie that you can buy in almost any convenience store—one of those giant cookies with fluffy pink frosting (sorry for putting that in your head). Notice that there are only 125 calories per serving. Wow, what if you really could eat an entire cookie of this size for only 125 calories? Now let's look at how many servings per container: four. Hmm, how many of us would buy one of these gargantuan cookies and eat only a fourth of it? I can't say that I would. Reading the serving size and servings per container takes almost no effort and can be extremely beneficial to your health.

*Calories.* This one is simple. Calories are listed (per serving, of course) right at the top of the food label under "Servings Per Container." Nutrition labels will also tell you how many calories come from fat per serving. This information is not as crucial, in my opinion, as it is easier to just look at the fat grams and try to stick to the rule of no more than 10 grams of fat per 300 calories; this will keep you in line with the current dietary advice of "Eat no more than 30 percent of total calories from fat" without having to carry a calculator around in your pocket.

*Nutrient Content & Percent Daily Value.* There are many nutrients in the foods we eat. However, current labels show only the nutrients that are most relevant to our health concerns today. Sugar, fat, saturated fat, cholesterol, and sodium are listed because they tend to be consumed in excess. Fiber, iron, calcium, and vitamins A and C tend to be the nutrients we don't get enough of. Fat, carbohydrate, and protein are the macronutrients found in foods that supply calories, or energy, to the human body. Protein and carbohydrates each supply four calories per gram of food, and

## Nutrition Facts

Serving Size ¼ cookie (28.35g)
Servings Per Container 4

**Amount Per Serving**

| Calories 113 | Calories from Fat 50 |
|---|---|

| | % Daily Value* |
|---|---|
| Total Fat 6g | 9% |
| Saturated Fat 2g | 6% |
| Cholesterol 4mg | 2% |
| Sodium 65mg | 3% |
| Total Carbohydrate 15g | 5% |
| Dietary Fiber 0g | 0% |
| Sugars 9g | |
| Protein 2g | |

| Vitamin A 2% | Vitamin C 0% |
|---|---|
| Calcium 0% | Iron 1% |

*Percent Daily Values are based on a 2,000 calorie diet. Your daily values may be higher or lower depending on your caloric needs:

| | Calories | 2,000 | 2,500 |
|---|---|---|---|
| Total Fat | Less Than | 65g | 80g |
| Saturated Fat | Less Than | 20g | 25g |
| Cholesterol | Less Than | 300mg | 300mg |
| Sodium | Less Than | 2,400mg | 2,400mg |
| Total Carbohydrate | | 300g | 375g |
| Dietary Fiber | | 25g | 30g |

Calories per gram:
Fat 9 • Carbohydrate 4 • Protein 4

fat provides nine (more than double) calories per gram of food. Alcohol also provides seven calories per gram. If any of the above nutrients are not on a food label, it is because the amount contained in one serving of the food is insignificant. Some foods will show more nutrients, specifically if a food has been fortified; however, showing other vitamins and minerals is voluntary for food manufacturers. It is also important to remember that "Percent Daily Value" is meant to show how a food fits into an overall daily diet; these values are based on a 2,000-calorie diet. Your personal needs may be higher or lower. I look at it as an opportunity to compare nutrients in a single food. For example, a look at the cookie label on page 29 shows that that particular food is too high in fat, sugar, and saturated fat, and too low in calcium and iron—regardless of what your personal calorie needs may be. We have begun to see unhealthy trans fat on the label, and even healthy monounsaturated fats.

*Ingredients.* The ingredient list is kind of like a recipe; it tells you what is in the food you are about to eat. One great thing about this section of the label is that the ingredients present in the highest amount (by weight) are listed first, and the list continues in descending order. So if sugar or oil is listed within the first couple of ingredients, you know that the food is going to be high in sugar or oil. With names like L-cysteine monohydrochloride, the ingredient list can sometimes be hard to read. I simply look through the first five or so ingredients and look for whole, natural ingredients rather than things like "partially hydrogenated vegetable oil"—which is essentially unhealthy trans fat. We will talk about partially hydrogenated oils and trans fats later in the chapter.

*Label Terms.* If you have ever walked through a grocery store, you've had a chance to decipher such label lingo as "Fat Free," "Cholesterol Free," "Reduced Sodium," "No Added Sugar," "Good Source of Fiber," or even the general term "Healthy." Only a handful of claims are actually approved for labels; things like "Low-Carb" have no established government guidelines. I will spare you the time and detail of what claim means what. Even as a dietitian, I don't find this topic all that interesting. I simply prefer to flip the container over and take a quick glance at the label. For example, if I am looking at a product claiming to be low-fat, I compare the label of the regular-fat product to that of the low-fat product. I look at the calories per serving (some low-fat products have the same number of, if not more, calories per serving) and the fat grams per serving to see just how much fat has really been cut out. This may seem time-consuming, but it really takes only about five seconds, and it helps you learn so much more about what you are putting into your body, rather than picking something up just because it claims to be "fat free."

My hope is that you at least become aware of what is on the label and start paying attention to the nutrient amounts in the foods you usually eat. After all, you have to eat several times a day, every single day. So learning a little here and there as you wander through the grocery store (or better yet, look through your own cupboard) will benefit you for the rest of your life.

## Portion Control

The day my husband brought home a 64-ounce refillable mug that he bought at a gas station, I almost cried. My mind quickly began calculating the number of calories a person could mindlessly drink in a short period of time (it's 833 for a non-diet soda). Then my husband informed me that he bought the mug to fill with water! Although I was relieved, I couldn't help but wonder, "What is the point of such an astronomically sized mug?" The word *supersized* may be one of the most recognized terms in our society today. Although it is common to relate this word strictly to fast food, we also have a portion-contortion problem with bakeries, bagel shops, donut shops, corner markets, dine-in restaurants, ice-cream shops, gas stations (most of these examples don't carry a food label, which compounds the problem), and even packaged foods. Our society has a giant disconnect in this area, and it runs all the way through our food supply. When I say "shrink serving sizes," that doesn't mean just when you eat out; it is something to think about every time you put something into your mouth.

Have you ever read the nutrition label of a "fat-free" nonstick cooking spray? If so, you surely noticed the miniscule serving size of a third-of-a-second spray. Granted, we rarely load up on massive doses of cooking spray, but doesn't the serving size seem unexpectedly small? To help you understand the importance of portion sizes, the next few pages provide pictures of commonly eaten portions versus recommended portions for everyday foods. There are also pictures of additionally recommended portion sizes for common foods. Portion sizes are so important to our long-term health that this is something I hope you will never forget.

# Eat Sensibly

| Recommended | Commonly Served |
|:---:|:---:|

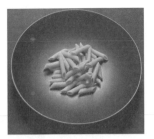

1 cup pasta

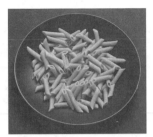

3 cups pasta

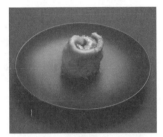

2 oz. cinnamon roll

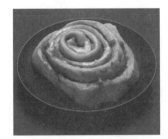

1 lb. cinamon roll

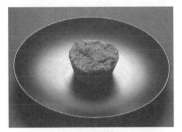

2 oz. muffin

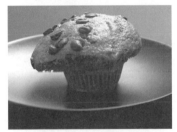

6 oz. muffin

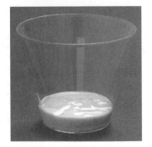

2 Tbsp. salad dressing

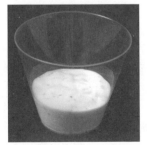

¼ cup salad dressing

# Step 2

| Recommended | Commonly Served |
|---|---|

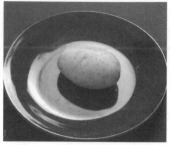

6 oz. potato

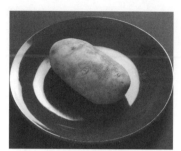

12 oz. potato

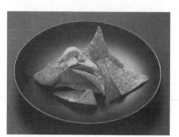

1 oz. chips

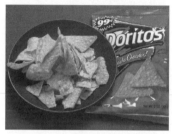

3 oz. chips

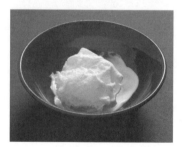

½ cup ice cream

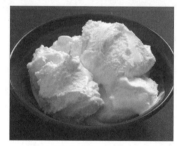

1½ cups ice cream

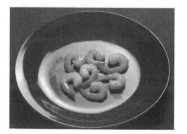

7 shrimp

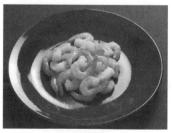

20 shrimp

[ 34 ]

## Additional Recommended Portions

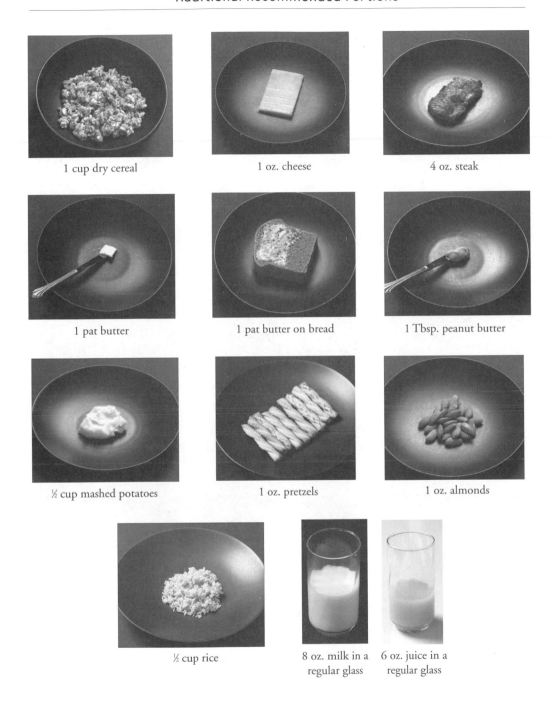

1 cup dry cereal

1 oz. cheese

4 oz. steak

1 pat butter

1 pat butter on bread

1 Tbsp. peanut butter

½ cup mashed potatoes

1 oz. pretzels

1 oz. almonds

½ cup rice

8 oz. milk in a regular glass

6 oz. juice in a regular glass

Now compare the following pictures: the amount for each of the foods shown provides 100 calories. So you could have two bites of chocolate vs. two cups of watermelon vs. three cups of plain popcorn.

## Which snack would you choose for 100 calories?

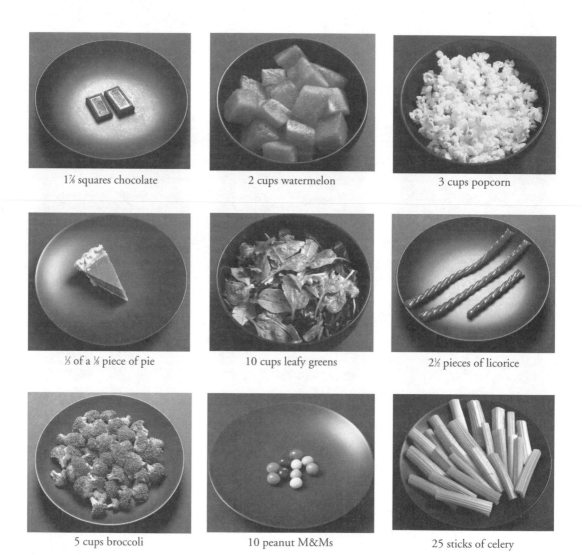

1⅞ squares chocolate      2 cups watermelon      3 cups popcorn

⅓ of a ⅛ piece of pie      10 cups leafy greens      2½ pieces of licorice

5 cups broccoli      10 peanut M&Ms      25 sticks of celery

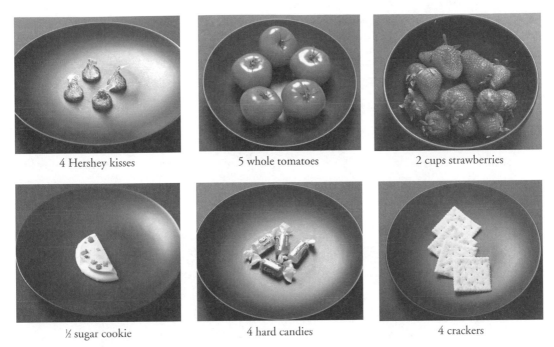

4 Hershey kisses      5 whole tomatoes      2 cups strawberries

½ sugar cookie      4 hard candies      4 crackers

We are blessed with a lot of food in this country, but that doesn't mean we have to eat it all at once. My judgment is that most of those servings look pretty small to you. In contrast, look at just one last picture:

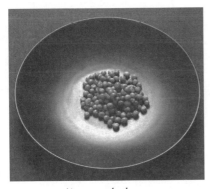

½ cup cooked peas

Does this picture look shockingly small, compared to what you usually eat or are served in a restaurant? Did the pictures of salad, fruit, or other vegetables look too small? The common answer is no. Isn't it ironic that we supersize the foods we should be eating less of, and not the foods we should be eating more of? Don't worry, all of us have fallen into this portion-control trap, and the time has come to climb out of it. Controlling portion sizes doesn't have to take a lot of time or effort. In fact, one of the best things you can do is take a couple of days over the next week and actually measure what you eat. Find out what one cup of milk looks like in *your* glass. Find out what one cup of cereal looks like in *your* bowl. I emphasize the word "your" because once you see the recommended portion in your own dishes, it will be easier to "eyeball" the correct portion size in the future. Taking time to measure a few foods before, during, or after meals will be an enlightening experience.

You may be thinking, "I am going to starve if I start eating these small portions!" However, there is good news. When you shrink your portion sizes, you get to eat more often! This is because a healthy metabolism thrives on small amounts of food eaten every two or three hours instead of heavy meals two or three times a day. As you learn to eat smaller portions more often, your blood sugar will become more stable, you will avoid fits of starvation and overeating, and your eating habits will become healthier.

## Healthy Eating Guidelines: Plant-Based Foods

In the midst of all the junk food in our society, I view plant foods—vegetables, fruits, whole grains, beans, and nuts—as almost medicinal. They are superior for our health. The scriptures confirm this (see D&C 89:10–11, 14), and current science confirms it too. Study after study has shown that plant-based foods fight the good fight against life-threatening disease, obesity, and deteriorating health. I believe in this so strongly that I can actually justify feeding my kids a slice of pizza if it's paired up with some vitamin A–loaded baby carrots, or maybe eating an occasional cheeseburger offset with a cup of vitamin C–rich strawberries. Plant-based foods offer a host of nutritional benefits but mainly supply carbohydrates (except nuts, which supply healthy fats) as a vital source of fuel. In the body, carbohydrates are metabolized into glucose, which is the preferred source of fuel for our muscles, heart, lungs, kidneys, and all other major organs and tissues. Even the brain is a "carbohydrate-dependent" organ! Carbohydrates have taken a bad rap in today's society—and I agree that the huge plates of pasta, gargantuan cinnamon rolls, teetering muffins, and all the other oversized, refined carbohydrate foods can go down with the ship. But healthy carbohydrate foods—plant-based foods like legumes, whole grains, fruits, and vegetables—shouldn't be on the "carbophobia" blacklist. These foods are full of vitamins, minerals, disease-reducing phytochemicals, fiber, carbohydrates, protein, and even healthy fats. But in 2003, 78 percent of the carbohydrate foods bought were refined, high-sugar products like soft drinks, sweetened grains, candy, and fruit drinks.[5] That means only 22 percent of carbohydrate foods bought were healthful ones like whole-wheat bread, cereal, pasta, and brown rice. Surely these numbers need to be reversed.

To help you incorporate "plant-based foods" into the fast-paced eating of real life, I've outlined the benefits of each plant-based food group (whole grains, fruits and vegetables, and legumes and nuts), how many servings you should strive for each day, practical tips for shopping and cooking, and even a top-ten choice for each food group.

## Whole Grains

Grains really are the staff of life and therefore should be the base of our diet. Whole grains contain many nutrients—essential vitamins, minerals, and fiber—that refined products do not. Besides that, replacing refined grains with whole grains can help you lose weight! Some may wonder, "What are refined grains, anyway?" It's ironic that grains are "whole" from the beginning (in fact, our ancestors knew of nothing other than whole grains). It is our own manmade technology that strips nutrients by removing the part of the seed or kernel that contains vitamins, minerals, fiber, and some protein, leaving the rest for us to eat. Granted, most refined grains are enriched with thiamin, riboflavin, niacin, and iron and are fortified (meaning that a nutrient not previously there has been added) with folic acid. But enrichment and fortification don't add up to the original nourishing quality of whole grains. Look at this table to get a clearer picture of why whole grains are better:

| NUTRIENT | WHITE BREAD | WHOLE WHEAT BREAD | WHITE RICE | BROWN RICE |
|---|---|---|---|---|
| Fiber (g) | .7 | 2 | 1 | 3.5 |
| Protein (g) | 2 | 2.8 | 3.4 | 5 |
| Potassium (mg) | 28 | 71 | 7 | 84 |
| Magnesium (mg) | 7 | 24 | 8 | 84 |
| Phosphorus (mg) | 28 | 65 | 23 | 162 |
| Vitamin B6 (mg) | .02 | .05 | .02 | .30 |
| Vitamin E (mg) | .06 | .09 | .02 | .06 |
| Zinc (mg) | .21 | .55 | .40 | 1.23 |
| Copper (mg) | .07 | .08 | .10 | .20 |

*Note: This chart does not reflect all the nutrients in specified foods; it reflects only the nutrients found in higher amounts in whole grains. Source: USDA Agricultural Research Service Nutrient Database for Standard Reference, Release 17.*

## *How Many Servings?*

Strive to eat at least three one-ounce servings of whole-grain foods per day. One serving equals half a cup of cooked brown rice, pasta, or cereal; one ounce (½ cup cooked) dry pasta or rice; one slice of bread; or one cup of ready-to-eat cereal.

## *Helpful Tips*

Read the label. Look for foods with at least three grams of fiber per serving. Also, take a second to review the ingredient list, looking for things like 100% whole-wheat or whole-grain flour, oats, or other grains that use the word "whole." Don't be fooled by "wheat flour" or "enriched flour" as they are not whole grains, but they are common ingredients. Sugars, fats, and oils should be toward the bottom of the ingredient list, or better yet, not there at all.

To help you get started with replacing those refined grains with more nutritious whole grains, here's your top-ten list for whole grains. Each list takes into consideration the foods that are highest in nutrients yet are realistically consumable (sometimes the highest-rated foods are those most of us never buy, let alone know how to cook).

*Top Ten Whole Grains*

1. 100 percent whole-wheat bread
2. Whole-wheat spaghetti or pasta
3. Brown rice
4. Old-fashioned rolled oats (or instant regular oatmeal)
5. High-fiber cereal (at least 5 grams of fiber per serving). Examples: All Bran®, Raisin Bran, Shredded Wheat, Grape Nuts®, Kashi® Go Lean
6. Wild rice
7. Bulgur (cracked wheat; this is simply a cleaned, precooked, dried, and ground form of whole wheat that can be used in place of rice; in stews, salads, casseroles, and baked goods; or as a breakfast cereal.)
8. Barley
9. Kashi® Pilaf hot cereal (this is a great hot cereal that can be eaten at any meal. It contains healthy grains that we don't often eat or know how to cook, such as barley, triticale, buckwheat, whole rye, and whole hard red winter wheat)
10. Popcorn (not butter-coated movie popcorn but plain old-fashioned popcorn.)

## Fruits and Vegetables

I know, I know; you've heard it a thousand times before: Eat your vegetables. Contrary to popular belief, dietitians don't tell you to eat more vegetables just to make your life more difficult. A lot of science stands behind this common but often ignored advice. A meager 22 percent of us actually eat five small servings of fruits and vegetables each day.[6]

Fruits and vegetables are one of the most widely studied food groups in health research. Fruit and vegetable intake has been studied in many types of diseases—all the way from cancer to cataracts to obesity. In the human body, oxidative stress is a major contributor to most disease processes. I like to think of oxidative stress as our own "metabolic rust" that can be a result of poor dietary habits, excessive exercise, aging, environmental factors, or even normal metabolism. Oxidative stress is also what creates our need for antioxidants consumed through food or supplements. In all practicality, antioxidants help gobble up the damaging metabolic rust (or oxidants) in our bodies. Antioxidants aren't another type of nutrient to worry about—they are actually simple vitamins and minerals like vitamin C, vitamin A, vitamin E, and selenium. Not only are fruits and vegetables great sources of antioxidants, but fruits and vegetables are also packed with phytochemicals, essential vitamins, minerals, and fiber.

*How Many Servings?*

Start by aiming to eat three servings of vegetables and two servings of fruit. After you accomplish that, strive for four to five servings of vegetables and three to four servings of fruit. One serving equals one medium piece of fresh fruit or vegetable (like one medium apple); half a cup of cooked, canned, or fresh fruit or vegetable; one cup of leafy greens; or half a cup of 100 percent juice. These serving sizes are actually quite small, so it is much easier than you think to build up to the recommended seven to nine daily servings of fruits and vegetables.

*Helpful Tips*

- Go for color. Green, orange, red, and yellow are great colors to look for as you shop. For example, the rich green color of spinach helps you pick the food with more nutrients as opposed to the drab light-green color of iceberg lettuce.
- Buy fresh. Yes, fresh is always better, but frozen is good too. If you must choose a canned vegetable, remember that canned foods have higher sodium content.

- Try smoothies. Even if you don't like fruit, you'll probably enjoy these. Blend fresh berries, bananas, frozen fruit, yogurt, or even orange juice for a tasty, nutritious treat. You can even make a large batch, freeze half, and then enjoy the other half later. Smoothies can have a lot of calories, so keep portion size to 8 ounces or less.

- Make salads exciting. Promise yourself right now that you will never again make a pale-green salad with croutons and buckets of salad dressing. Instead, use dark green lettuces and chunks of fresh vegetables (lots and lots!), such as carrots, tomatoes, cucumbers, broccoli, peppers, and sugar-snap peas.

- Cut up fruits or veggies in advance. Cut up your melons, wash your grapes, slice your tomatoes, or even buy pre-cut fruits and veggies. How can you refuse a bite of delicious fruit or vegetable when it is sitting right there in your refrigerator—washed, cut, and ready to eat?

- Experiment. Try one new fruit or vegetable each month. You can find quick and easy recipes online or even right at the grocery store! Check out the official 5-A-Day website for fun new ideas: www.5aday.com.

- Keep apples, pears, oranges, or dried fruit in your car, just to help you drive past the "drive-through" in a fit of hunger. Snacking on an apple or piece of fruit will help you make it through the traffic so you can eat something healthier at home.

- Use salsa. Try it on baked potatoes, as a veggie dip, or, yes, even with a few tortilla chips.

*Top Ten Fruits*

1. Strawberries
2. Kiwifruit
3. Grapefruit
4. Oranges
5. Cantaloupe

6. Watermelon
7. Raspberries
8. Mango or papaya
9. Banana
10. Apple

*Top Ten Vegetables*

1. Spinach, collard greens, kale, or swiss chard
2. Broccoli
3. Carrots
4. Peppers
5. Sweet potato
6. Peas
7. Asparagus
8. Cauliflower
9. Celery
10. Corn

## Legumes

What are legumes anyway? Legumes are basically beans, peas, or lentils—they have a pod that splits on two sides to reveal a fruit or seed. Legumes are unique because, like fruits and vegetables, they contain vitamins, minerals, phytochemicals, and fiber; but, like meat, they are a good source of protein and therefore a healthy alternative to meat. Legumes are also a good source of complex carbohydrates—the kind that take longer to digest and promote healthy metabolism. Unfortunately, beans are underappreciated. They seem to have the reputation for causing gas (and they can!). However, beans are so nutritious that it's a shame to not eat them when the side-effects are so easily avoidable. To get rid of the gas-producing carbohydrates, simply drain the liquid from the can, rinse the canned beans thoroughly with water, and then cook thoroughly. Or for dried beans, soak overnight, discard the water, rinse thoroughly, cool in fresh water until soft, and throw into your favorite dish. Beans are a great alternative to meat and blend right in with casseroles, stews or soups, grain dishes, ethnic dishes, or even your favorite pasta.

*How Many Servings?*

You don't have to eat legumes every day, but you should strive for at least four servings per week. One serving is only half a cup of cooked beans, peas, or lentils.

*Helpful Tips*

- Soak beans to reduce cooking time by up to one half. Fill a pot with room-temperature water and soak for at least four hours or overnight. (If you're pressed for time, boil some water, remove from heat, and soak beans one to three hours.) Remember to choose a pot big enough, because beans will expand. Then discard the water, rinse the beans well, and cook them in fresh water.

- When cooking beans, use approximately six cups of water to each pound of dry beans. Don't add salt or acidic foods (like tomatoes) until the end of cooking, as they can toughen the beans and prolong the cooking time.

- Add a tiny bit of cooking oil to the boiling water to keep the beans from foaming as they cook.

- If you're on the run (like me), use canned, precooked beans.

- Add beans to soups, salads, stews, casseroles, or pasta dishes.

- Use beans as a baked-potato topper.

- Try filling a whole-wheat tortilla with beans and salsa or some low-fat cheese.

*Top Ten Legumes*

1. Kidney beans
2. Black beans
3. Garbanzo beans
4. Split green peas
5. Pinto beans
6. Lentils
7. Navy beans
8. White beans
9. Soybeans
10. Lima beans

## Nuts

When you think of nuts, what comes to mind? Salty peanuts? Most people don't realize that nuts offer a wealth of good nutrition. Although nuts are very healthful, the key is to eat raw or dry-roasted, unsalted nuts *in moderation.* Nuts are a great source of healthy monounsaturated and Omega-3 fats, protein, fiber, magnesium, and vitamin E. The downside is that nuts are also packed with calories. An ounce of nuts (a small handful in most cases) can pack almost 200 calories, so although it is important to make nuts a regular part of your diet, they should be consumed in small portions and should replace other less-healthy foods (like potato chips, for example). Common tree nuts such as almonds, walnuts, pecans, hazelnuts, pistachios, and macadamias have all been shown to modestly lower cholesterol.[7] Nuts have proven so healthful that the Food and Drug Administration has authorized a qualified health claim for them: "Scientific evidence suggests but does not prove that eating 1.5 ounces per day of most nuts (almonds, hazelnuts, pecans, pistachios, walnuts) as part of a diet low in saturated fat and cholesterol may reduce the risk of heart disease."[8] Nuts also offer antioxidant and anti–blood-clotting properties. Although nuts have many amazing properties, they can also be extremely allergenic. Peanuts account for most allergies, and the allergic response can be life threatening.[9] So be careful when adding them as a new food—especially for children.

*How Many Servings?*

Strive to eat 1 to 1½ ounces (one to two handfuls) at least four times per week. If you have high cholesterol or heart disease, strive to eat 1.5 to 2 ounces every day—as a substitution for other foods, and not as an addition to an already calorie-adequate diet. And just to set the record straight, I did not just recommend that you eat a handful of Peanut M&Ms every day. Sorry! These recommendations are for dry-roasted or raw nuts, unsalted.

*Helpful Tips*

- To get more flavor out of nuts, toast them in a 350-degree oven for about five minutes— then use the nuts as a topping or stirred into your favorite recipes.
- Add nuts to any green salad, cooked vegetables (like green beans), or your favorite cereal.

- Keep nuts around the house or office for a quick and nutritious snack (only one handful please!).
- Add a dollop or two of low-fat sour cream or Cool Whip to a bowl of fresh berries and top with your favorite nuts.
- Throw nuts into your favorite fruit salad.

*Top Ten Nuts*

1. Almonds
2. Pecans
3. Walnuts
4. Hazelnuts
5. Pistachios
6. Macadamias
7. Peanuts
8. Cashews
9. Pine nuts
10. Beechnuts

## Fiber

We've talked about many of the positive benefits of plant-based foods. However, plant-based foods offer one more giant bonus: fiber. Fiber is a very broad term for compounds of plant origin that your body cannot digest. Since fiber is not something your body uses for energy, it is technically not a nutrient, but it is something that promotes good health in many other ways. Fiber plays a key role in our health: (1) it stimulates chewing, saliva flow, and secretion of gastric juices; (2) it fills the stomach and leads to a feeling of fullness; (3) it "normalizes" bowel function; (4) it delays stomach emptying and therefore slows the rate of digestion and absorption of nutrients; and (5) it lowers serum cholesterol and the rate of glucose (carbohydrate or sugar) absorption, which helps control diabetes and heart disease.[10] Fiber also helps fight cancer and weight gain. Fibrous foods take longer to chew and eat, allowing your brain to send the "I'm full" signal to help you avoid overeating.

It shouldn't come as a big surprise to hear that Americans don't consume enough fiber—currently the average intake is only 15 grams per day.[11] However, we need to consume 25 to 35 grams per day. There are two unique kinds of fiber: soluble and insoluble. Soluble fibers are protective because they bind fatty substances and can lower cholesterol levels. Soluble fibers are found in foods like oats, legumes, apples, and oranges. Insoluble fibers are digestive aids. They add bulk and softness to stools, promote regularity, and help prevent constipation. Insoluble fibers are found in whole-wheat products, vegetables, and seeds. Both kinds of fiber are good for you. The bottom line is that plant-based foods offer a good blend of soluble and insoluble fiber. So simply by eating a variety of whole grains, fruits, vegetables, beans, and nuts, you will get ample amounts of both kinds of fiber.

I could go on for pages about how good fiber is for our health, but the question on everybody's mind is "What will fiber do to my bowels?" People are often afraid that fiber will cause constipation, diarrhea, or intestinal gas. The interesting thing about fiber, especially insoluble fiber, is that whatever the ailment is, constipation or diarrhea, fiber works to "normalize" the bowels. If you have constipation, fiber can help soften the stool. If you have diarrhea, fiber can help slow things down. However, intestinal gas is a common side effect as a result of drastic changes in fiber consumption. For example, if you currently eat very little fiber (less than 10 grams per day) and you suddenly up your fiber intake to 30 grams a day, you may have some intestinal problems because the fiber was added into your diet too quickly. Keep in mind that some people experience no side effects from added fiber. Here are some quick tips to help you add fiber into your diet without causing excessive intestinal side effects:

- Add fiber gradually to the diet. Aim to replace one refined grain or high-fat food with a high-fiber food every few days. The goal is to increase fiber by about 5 grams every few days or maybe even every week until you're consuming about 30 grams per day.
- Try cooked or canned fruits, vegetables, and beans because they may be better tolerated. Fresh is always best, but starting this way is just fine.

- Drink plenty of fluids—at least 8 to 10 glasses per day. (Sorry, caffeinated beverages don't count because they have a diuretic effect and cause water loss.)

Remember that you can get too much of a good thing. Eating more than 50 grams of fiber per day can lead to nutrient absorption and digestive problems.

Here are some quick and easy ways to add fiber to your diet:

- Choose whole-grain breads, cereal, rice, or pasta over the white, refined versions. Take a quick second to check the nutrition label for fiber. If you ever purchase a loaf of "brown" bread and it has less than one gram of fiber per slice, you likely just purchased bread made with a combination of refined white flour, wheat flour, and a little caramel coloring.

- Choose fruits with edible skins or seeds such as apples, pears, peaches, strawberries, kiwis, and raspberries.

- Eat the skin on your baked potato, and leave the skin on when mashing potatoes.

- Have a salad full of chopped vegetables (like carrots, broccoli, tomatoes, peas, and cucumbers) every day if you can.

- Use whole-grain flours when cooking. Simply substitute whole-grain flour for half of the white flour. (Of course, going with all whole-grain flour is great too!)

- Use breakfast as a time to get regular fiber every day—choose oatmeal or another high-fiber cereal.

- Snack on raw veggies or fruits or plain popcorn.

- Eat foods in their most natural state. An apple with the peel has 3 grams of fiber, a peeled apple has 2.4 grams of fiber, a half cup of applesauce has 1.8 grams of fiber, and a cup of apple juice has .2 grams of fiber.[12]

- Replace refined foods or other snacks with whole grains, fruits, vegetables, beans, peas, and nuts.

# Fiber Content of Some Common Foods

| FOOD | PORTION | GRAMS of FIBER | FOOD | PORTION | GRAMS of FIBER |
|---|---|---|---|---|---|
| **Breads** | | | **Vegetables** | | |
| White | 1 slice | 0.6 | Summer Squash | 1 cup | 1.2 |
| Sourdough | 1 slice | 1.0 | Tomato | 1 medium | 1.4 |
| Wheat | 1 slice | 1.1 | Winter Squash | 1 cup | 2.1 |
| Wheat Bran | 1 slice | 1.4 | Broccoli | 1 cup | 2.3 |
| 7-Grain | 1 slice | 1.7 | Carrots | 1 cup | 3.6 |
| Whole Wheat | 1 slice | 1.9 | Green Beans | 1 cup | 3.7 |
| | | | Corn—yellow | 1 cup | 4.0 |
| **Cereals** | | | Potato—with skin | 1 medium | 4.6 |
| Corn Flakes | 1 cup | 0.7 | Artichoke | 1 medium | 6.9 |
| Lucky Charms | 1 cup | 1.5 | | | |
| Cheerios | 1 cup | 3.6 | **Pasta** | | |
| Total, Whole Grain | 1 cup | 3.6 | Macaroni—enriched | 1 cup | 1.8 |
| Shredded Wheat Bran | 1 cup | 6.3 | Spaghetti | 1 cup | 2.4 |
| Raisin Bran | 1 cup | 7.3 | Whole-Wheat Spaghetti | 1 cup | 6.3 |
| All-Bran Buds | 1 cup | 38.7 | | | |
| | | | **Legumes** | | |
| **Rice** | | | Lima Beans | 1 cup | 9.0 |
| White | ½ cup | 0.6 | Kidney Beans | 1 cup | 11.3 |
| Mexican | ½ cup | 2.2 | Garbanzo Beans | 1 cup | 12.5 |
| Spanish | ½ cup | 3.0 | Black Beans | 1 cup | 15.0 |
| Wild | ½ cup | 3.0 | Pinto Beans | 1 cup | 15.4 |
| Brown | ½ cup | 3.5 | Lentils | 1 cup | 15.6 |
| | | | Navy Beans | 1 cup | 19.1 |
| **Fruits** | | | | | |
| Grapes | 1 cup | 0.8 | **Nuts** | | |
| Banana | 1 medium | 3.1 | Cashews | 1 ounce | 0.9 |
| Apple | 1 medium | 3.3 | Walnuts | 1 ounce | 1.9 |
| Strawberries—sliced | 1 cup | 3.3 | Brazils | 1 ounce | 2.1 |
| Orange | 1 medium | 3.4 | Pecans | 1 ounce | 2.7 |
| Raspberries | 1 cup | 8.0 | Pistachios | 1 ounce | 2.9 |
| Avocado—California | 1 medium | 8.5 | Almonds | 1 ounce | 3.3 |

*Source: USDA Agricultural Research Service Nutrient Database for Standard Reference, Release 17.*

It may seem as if you have to make drastic changes in your diet to get your fiber intake up to par, but in reality it is easy. You don't have to eat huge amounts of healthy foods; you just have to make wiser everyday choices.

Some may wonder if they can simply take a pill or a powder for fiber and still enjoy their light and fluffy white bread. Unfortunately, most pills offer only a fraction of the fiber you really need, and powders (and pills) don't offer the "total package" that high-fiber foods do—like essential vitamins and minerals. It is okay to take a fiber pill or powder once in a while to relieve constipation, but you shouldn't use fiber pills, powder, or laxatives regularly because your bowels can become dependent on them.

## The Bottom Line: Plant-Based Foods

Plant-based foods are essential for good health, disease prevention, and weight control. To make plant-based foods the base of your diet:

1. Eat at least three servings of vegetables (remember, portion sizes are actually quite small—a half cup cooked) and two servings of fruits each day—and remember that more is better!
2. Eat at least three servings of whole grains each day.
3. Each week, eat at least four servings of beans, peas, or lentils.
4. Eat one ounce of nuts (a small handful) at least four times per week; if you have high cholesterol or heart disease, eat one to two ounces of nuts each day.
5. Try to get 25 to 35 grams of fiber per day. If you experience digestive problems, add fiber slowly to your diet.

Not all foods are created equal, so it is important to shake up your diet and get plenty of variety in the foods you eat. Choosing foods with fiber will generally lead you to the foods that are lower in fat and cholesterol (and even calories) and higher in phytochemicals, vitamins, and minerals.

## Healthy Fats

"Fat" and "healthy" in the same phrase? Does that sound strange to you? If you're like most Americans, you assume that all fat is evil and wreaks havoc on your health. You might also assume that most of America went on a low-fat diet (remember the Snackwells craze?) in the late 1980s and 1990s. We didn't. And currently, most of us eat too much of the unhealthy fats and possibly not enough of the healthy fats.

There are several different kinds of dietary fat, and they all play different roles in our health. Here are some of the terms that relate to dietary fat and our health:

*Fat:* Fat is actually a nutrient—your body can't survive without it. Fat supplies the body with essential fatty acids and helps with the absorption of the fat-soluble vitamins A, D, E, and K. Fat also supplies our bodies with energy. Even though fat is essential for our bodies, we tend to consume too much. It takes only 15 to 25 grams of dietary fat from mixed sources to meet the minimum requirement.[13] Most of us gobble up 65 to 90 grams of fat every day.[14] Dietary fats can be classified into four main categories: saturated fat, polyunsaturated fat, monounsaturated fat, and trans fat.

*Saturated Fat:* The more saturated a fat is, the more solid it is at room temperature (the exception is coconut oil, which is very saturated but can be liquid at mildly warm temperatures). Saturated fat comes from animal sources such as meat, poultry, milk, cheese, butter, and lard, and from tropical oils such as coconut, palm, and palm kernel oil. You might think that dietary cholesterol raises blood cholesterol, but actually saturated fat is the leading contributor to high blood cholesterol levels!

*Polyunsaturated Fat:* Polyunsaturated fats are found in fish, vegetable oils, flaxseed, and nuts. Polyunsaturated fats may help improve blood cholesterol levels when substituted for saturated fat in the diet. You may have heard about "Omega-3" (also referred to as marine-derived "EPA" and "DHA" and plant-derived "ALA") and "Omega-6" fats. Both of these are polyunsaturated fats, and they are the only two types of fatty acids that are essential for human health. However, Omega-3 fats are gaining a lot of positive attention because they seem to protect the heart and overall health. Omega-3 fats help regulate heartbeat and help reduce harmful arrhythmias, blood clots, and inflammation. Omega-3 fats are found in fatty cold-water fish, canola oil, liquid soybean oil (not the hydrogenated kind found in processed foods), walnuts, and ground flaxseed or flaxseed oil. Omega-6 fats are found in many processed foods and most vegetable oils like corn, sunflower, and sesame oil. Most of us get plenty of Omega-6 fats because we eat a lot of processed foods that use corn, hydrogenated soybean, or hydrogenated cottonseed oils as the main source of fat. Overall, we need to get more Omega-3 fats from fish (like salmon), nuts, canola oil, or flaxseed, and we need to eat less fat from processed foods, baked goods, and salty snacks. And even though some fat is essential, that doesn't mean it's okay to eat a pint of ice cream (which is full of nonessential saturated fat) every night—you only need about a tablespoon per day of canola oil to meet your essential fatty acid needs.

*Monounsaturated Fat:* Monounsaturated fats, along with Omega-3 fats, are some the healthiest fats we can eat. They are found in canola, olive, and safflower oil, and I use the acronym COS to help me remember this. (Yes, this is how I got through college.) There is also a chart on page 59 to help you diciper which oils are healthiest. Monounsaturated fats are also found in avocados, nuts, and peanut butter (preferably the natural, nonhydrogenated, grainy peanut butter). Recent research shows that replacing saturated fat with monounsaturated fat is quite beneficial for heart health. In fact, monounsaturated fats seem to reduce LDL (the "bad" cholesterol) levels while at the same time keeping the HDL ("good" cholesterol) levels stable.

*Trans Fat:* Trans fats are the result of food manufacturers taking polyunsaturated fats (like corn, soybean, and cottonseed oils) that are liquid at room temperature and "hydrogenating" them (adding hydrogen atoms) to make them more solid, shelf stable, and suitable for frying foods. Trans fats are found in stick margarine, shortening, bakery goods, snack foods, some hydrogenated peanut butters, and many processed foods. However, about 20 percent of the trans fat we eat comes from natural sources like milk and meat.[15] Trans fats are not healthy. They can raise bad cholesterol, which, of course, is bad. And they can lower good cholesterol, which is very bad. However, the American diet is about five times higher in saturated fat than in trans fat. So even though trans fat is widespread in our food supply, it occurs in much smaller amounts.[16] Instead of trying to figure out which one is worse, the bottom line is simple: eat less of both.

Any time you see "partially hydrogenated vegetable oil" or "hydrogenated vegetable oil" in the first two or three ingredients on a food label, take it as a sign that the food contains trans fat. A new FDA regulation will require trans fat grams per serving to be listed on food labels starting in January 2006. This will likely prompt the food industry to choose healthier oils in food production, which is great news for all of us who need to take better care of our hearts.

*Cholesterol:* Cholesterol is not a fat; it is a waxy, fat-like substance. Our bodies naturally produce cholesterol. In fact, only a third of the cholesterol found in our body is from dietary sources—our bodies naturally make the other two-thirds. Cholesterol plays an important role in the synthesis of bile acids, steroid hormones (like estrogen and progesterone), and vitamin D, and it is a key component in the structure of our cell membranes. Cholesterol from food is found only in animal products like egg yolks, butter, and meat. It is not found in anything plant-based like vegetable oil, margarine, grains, nuts, fruits, or vegetables. (So I keep thinking that someone should write to the manufacturers of all of those plant-based products that tout "no cholesterol" on their products and let them know that their product never had any cholesterol in the first place!)

*Triglycerides:* Simply put, "triglyceride" is the scientific name for 95 percent of the fat in our diet. In food we just call it fat, but in the body we call it a triglyceride. Testing blood triglyceride levels is very common. High levels of triglycerides in your blood are unhealthy for your body. Surprisingly, high triglyceride levels are not always caused by eating too much fat; eating too many refined carbohydrates is also a major cause. Obesity, diabetes, and other chronic medical conditions can also contribute to high triglyceride levels. Triglycerides are a highly concentrated source of energy. Most stored body fat is in the form of triglycerides. So when we assume that all that lovely body fat is useless, that really is not true; it is a bundle of energy just waiting to be used up! Moreover, achieving and maintaining a healthy weight is one of the best ways to lower triglyceride levels. (Yep, that's just another reason to get moving.)

*HDL-cholesterol:* HDL stands for High Density Lipoprotein. HDL is not in the food we eat; it is a "transporter" of cholesterol in our bodies. HDL is known as the "good" cholesterol because it carries cholesterol away from body tissues, helping to excrete cholesterol from the body. HDL is protective. We can increase our HDL levels by getting regular exercise (yes, there's another reason) and by losing excess weight.

*LDL-cholesterol:* LDL stands for Low Density Lipoprotein. LDL also is not in the food we eat; LDL functions as the primary transporter of cholesterol in our body. LDL is known as the "bad" cholesterol because it slyly and efficiently delivers cholesterol to our body tissues and can oxidize, or form deposits, on our artery walls or other blood vessels. High levels of LDL in the blood are a major risk factor for heart disease. Eating too much saturated or trans fat, even more so than cholestrerol, is what raises our LDL cholesterol to risky levels.

## How Much Fat Should We Eat?

The general guideline is to eat no more than 30 percent of your daily calories from fat. You should consume no more than 10 percent (7 percent if you have heart disease) of your calories from harmful saturated and trans fat. For a person on a 2,000-calorie-per-day diet, that means no more than 65 grams of fat per day, and no more than 15 to 22 grams of the unhealthy saturated or trans fat per day. A 2.5-cup restaurant serving of fettuccine alfredo packs 48 grams of unhealthy saturated fat (oh, and 1,500 calories to boot). A traditional American cheeseburger and french fries can easily slither 20 to 25 grams of unhealthy saturated fat into our veins. See why we have problems?

An easy way to monitor your fat intake is to eat no more than 10 grams of fat per 300 calories. For optimal health, the majority of these fat calories should come from vegetable oils (non-hydrogenated), nuts, avocados, natural peanut butter, flaxseed, or seafood. However healthy these fats may be, we still tend to eat too much fat. So make it a point to *replace*—not add—unhealthy fats or processed foods with healthy ones. For example, just because olive oil is healthful doesn't mean you need to drench your salad in oil. Two tablespoons of olive oil has 240 calories, so it should still be used sparingly. Each gram of fat still packs 9 calories—more than double that of carbohydrates or protein.

We should also try to eat less than 300 milligrams of cholesterol per day. Cholesterol is in its own league. It doesn't provide calories, but it does affect our health. One egg yolk has 215 milligrams of cholesterol. So it is wise to consume no more than four egg yolks per week. However, you can still enjoy eggs; just try to use two egg whites to one yolk—or try an egg substitute.

## Tips for Decreasing Fat Intake

Here are some tips to help you decrease your intake of unhealthy fats and moderate your intake of healthy fats:

- Buy and order the leanest possible cuts of meat: reduced-fat ground beef, sirloin steak, or filet mignon (skip the bacon).

- Trim visible fat from meat before and even after cooking.

- Remove the skin from poultry. Enjoy grilled or baked skinless chicken breasts.

- Skip fried chicken breasts, strips, or nuggets. You can still buy breaded chicken, but you should bake it in the oven for a crisp, trans-fat-free piece of meat.

- Choose low-fat dairy products such as low-fat milk and low-fat yogurt.

- Go easy on all fats and oils: butter, margarine, cooking oil, salad dressings, sauces, and cream cheese. Remember, it doesn't take much fat to meet your needs for good health.

- Read food labels. Watch total fat, saturated fat, and—coming soon—trans fat.

- Balance high-fat foods with low-fat foods. A crisp salad with plenty of vegetables (not eggs, cheese, and meat) and a little salad dressing is the perfect example of balancing fat and calories.

- Buy a non-stick skillet so you can decrease the need for oil in cooking.

- If you eat out more than two times per week, save your fat grams for your meals! You will get plenty of fat, whether you want it or not, from most restaurant entrees. Balance those higher-fat meals by snacking on low-fat or fat-free foods: whole grains, fresh fruits, or raw vegetables.

- Ask for dressings, sauces, and gravies on the side.

- Experiment with fresh herbs or flavored vinegars to add flavor instead of drenching your food with butter, salt, and pepper.

- Watch portions. A serving of meat should be the approximate size and thickness of a deck of cards.

- Switch to canola or olive oil for cooking and salad dressings.

- Don't forget about all the wonderful foods you *can* eat: whole grains, fresh fruits, vegetables, nuts, lean meats, and low-fat dairy.

## One Last Question: Margarine or Butter?

Keeping up with science on the issue of whether to use margarine or butter could become a full-time job, but the current recommendation is to stick with soft-tub margarine made with one of the healthier oils. Butter is loaded with saturated fat. Stick margarine is vegetable oil turned solid. Remember, the more solid a food is, the more saturated (or trans) fat is in the food. Therefore, a soft-tub or liquid margarine is better for your health.

## The Bottom Line: Healthy Fats in Moderation

So remember, not all fat is bad. Fat is an essential part of our diet, a concentrated energy source, and a vital component to the human body—oh, and fat makes things taste delicious too!

Just remember to sort your fats and stick to the healthiest kinds:

- Cut down on saturated and trans fats from animal products and processed or fried foods.
- Try to eat more unsaturated fats from canola, olive, or other vegetable oils, and from avocados, nuts, or seafood.
- Try to eat more Omega-3 fatty acids from fish, walnuts, canola oil, or flaxseed.

One serving of healthy fat is approximately:

- One tablespoon of oil, salad dressing, peanut butter, or other side items and toppings.
- A fourth of an avocado.
- Two to three tablespoons of ground flaxseed.
- One tablespoon of flaxseed oil or fish oil.
- One ounce of nuts (a small handful).
- Six ounces of cooked salmon, trout, herring, or other fatty fish.

Use the chart below to help you sort the healthy fats from the unhealthy fats.

## Fatty Acid Composition of Common Oils & Fats*

| Healthy Plant Oils | | | |
|---|---|---|---|
| | Monounsaturated Fat (g) | Polyunsaturated Fat (g) | Saturated Fat (g) |
| Safflower oil** | 75 | 14 | 6 |
| Olive oil | 74 | 10 | 13 |
| Canola oil | 59 | 30 | 7 |
| Peanut oil | 46 | 32 | 17 |
| Sunflower oil | 45 | 45 | 10 |
| Sesame oil | 40 | 42 | 14 |
| Corn oil | 28 | 55 | 13 |
| Soybean oil | 23 | 58 | 14 |
| Canola-based soft-tub margarine | 18 | 43 | 11 |
| Unhealthy Saturated Oils and/or Trans Fats | | | |
| | Monounsaturated Fat (g) | Polyunsaturated Fat (g) | Saturated Fat (g) |
| Stick margarine* source of trans fat | 37 | 23 | 15 |
| Hydrogenated soybean and/or cottonseed oil* source of trans fat | 30 | 48 | 18 |
| Lard | 45 | 11 | 39 |
| Palm oil | 37 | 9 | 49 |
| Butter | 21 | 3 | 51 |
| Palm kernel oil | 11 | 16 | 82 |
| Coconut oil | 6 | 2 | 86 |

*Amount per 100 grams*

** *High-oleic safflower oil (highly monounsaturated) made up 85% of the 2004 crop according to Robert Reeves of the Institute of Shortening and Edible Oils*

*Source: USDA Agricultural Research Service Nutrient Database for Standard Reference, Release 17.*

Check this chart to see the amount of fat found in commonly consumed foods:

## DIETARY FAT IN COMMON FOODS

| FOOD | PORTION | FAT GRAMS |
|------|---------|-----------|
| Skim Milk | 1 cup | .45 |
| Whole Milk | 1 cup | 8.0 |
| Fried Chicken | 1 piece | 15 |
| Baked Chicken Breast | 1 piece | 3.0 |
| Shrimp | 3 ounce | 1.0 |
| Salmon | 3 ounce | 10.5 |
| Tuna | 3 ounce | 5.0 |
| Small Hamburger with Bun | 1 sandwich | 12 |
| Prime Rib | 3 ounce | 32 |
| Steak, Porterhouse | 3 ounce | 8 |
| Popcorn with Oil | 1 cup | 3 |
| Popcorn, Air-Popped | 1 cup | .35 |
| Brownie | 2-inch squared | 10 |
| Glazed Donut | Medium 3-3/4″ diameter | 14 |
| Chocolate Chip Cookie | Medium 2-1/4″ diameter | 3 |
| Potato Chips | 1 ounce bag | 10 |
| Cashews | 1 ounce | 13 |
| Ice-Cream | 1/2 cup | 8 |
| Candy Bar— Snickers | 2 ounce | 15 |
| French Fries | 114 grams medium | 22 |
| Pizza— Pepperoni | 113 grams 1 serving | 16 |

*Source: USDA Agricultural Research Service Nutrient Database for Standard Reference, Release 17.*

# Lean Meats and Other Protein-Rich Foods

Whether it's roasted, broiled, braised, stewed, smothered in gravy or ketchup (and often in cheese), or just plain cooked to sizzling perfection, Americans love their beef. When you think of an all-American meal, what comes to mind? Meat and potatoes, of course! Think of any traditional entrée in our society today—pizza, burgers, tacos, stews and soups, chili, kabobs, fajitas, fine cuts of beef, poultry, pork, lamb, or seafood, and even salads, sandwiches, and pasta dishes—it's all about meat. Meat does provide our bodies with essential protein, zinc, iron, and B vitamins. Vitamin B12 for example, is found only in animal products. However, we don't have to eat enormous portions of meat at every meal. And we don't have to eat enormous portions of meat every day. In fact, we don't *have* to eat meat at all. Other foods such as nuts or seeds, peanut butter, eggs, beans and other legumes, tofu, and soy or dairy products are great sources of the protein our bodies need to survive.

I am neither advocating nor discouraging vegetarianism. Whether you eat no meat, little meat, or all meat, any dietary habits that become too extreme and restrictive can be detrimental to your health. However, for those of us who do eat and enjoy meat, we need to eat smaller portions and aim to eat meat less often. If you currently eat meat at all three meals, you might set a goal to eat meat only once or twice each day. The scriptures, our past prophets, and even current, cutting-edge scientists agree—we need to associate the word "sparingly" with meat with much more zeal. You know the theory "If a little is good, a lot must be better"? First off, that statement is rarely true for any health-related concept, and second, that statement is certainly not true for meat. Meat is known to all as a good source of protein, and our bodies absolutely need protein to survive. However, as stated above, protein is found in many other foods. Protein serves as a major structural component in every cell in our bodies. Proteins also function as enzymes, membrane receptors, hormones, carriers of nutrients in the blood, and even antibodies that protect our bodies from bacteria and viruses. Protein is a busy nutrient; its unique function is to build and repair tissues and regulate body processes. If you aren't getting enough calories from carbohydrates and fat in the diet, protein can be used for energy—but that is not its primary role. During digestion, proteins are broken down into amino acids, the building blocks of life. Some amino acids are "essential" and some are termed "non-essential." Where one food may lack an essential amino acid, another food may provide ample amounts. Animal proteins like meat and eggs offer high-quality, highly-digestible essential amino acids. However, by enjoying a variety of plant-based foods, your diet can provide (or your body will manufacture from pieces here and there) all of the essential amino acids. Only those who are on very strict vegan diets (no dairy, eggs, or any animal product) or those who choose only raw, vegan foods may need to put a little extra planning into their diets to make sure they get adequate protein and all the essential amino acids.

The U.S. Recommended Dietary Allowance for protein for an average healthy adult is .8 grams per kilogram of body weight. That comes out to about 55 grams of protein for a 150-pound adult, or 67 grams of protein for a 185-pound adult. I have often heard it said (mostly in health clubs and fitness areas) that the U.S. RDA for protein is too low. However, the U.S. Food and Nutrition Board and the National Institute of Medicine issued a report in 2002 stating the new Daily Reference Intakes for energy, carbohydrates, fiber, fat, fatty acids, cholesterol, protein, and amino acids.[17] And guess what: The RDA for protein still holds at .8 grams per kilogram. Take comfort in knowing that, unlike other areas of nutrition (which sometimes feels like an "it's good for you, no, it's bad for you" cycle), the RDA for protein has remained constant. Besides, what does the government, which already has 1.3 trillion dollars in health-care costs to worry about, have to gain from sending a message that could cause nutritional deficiencies and medical problems? More health care costs?

Take a moment to compare the few sample menus below to see how easy it is to meet and even exceed your daily needs for protein:

## MENU #1: NO MEAT PRODUCTS

| FOOD | PROTEIN (GRAMS) |
|---|---|
| 1 cup corn flakes | 2 |
| ¾ cup low-fat milk | 6.75 |
| 1 medium banana | 1.3 |
| 1 cup orange juice | 2 |
| 1 ounce pretzels | 3 |
| 1 peanut butter and jam sandwich on wheat bread | 13.5 |
| 1 medium apple | 0.5 |
| 1 (6-oz.) container blueberry yogurt | 6.75 |
| 1 cup vegetarian chili | 12 |
| 5 saltine crackers | 1.5 |
| 1 cup low-fat milk | 9 |
| 1 cup baby carrots | 1.3 |

### TOTAL PROTEIN FOR DAY: 60 GRAMS

## MENU #2: TYPICAL AMERICAN DAY ON THE RUN

| FOOD | PROTEIN (GRAMS) |
|---|---|
| 2 scrambled eggs | 12.5 |
| 1 cup orange juice | 2 |
| 1 ounce pretzels | 3 |
| 1 double cheeseburger | 21 |
| 1 order medium French fries | 6 |
| 1 Snickers bar | 4.5 |
| 1 (6-oz.) grilled chicken breast | 53 |
| 1 cup mashed potatoes | 5.5 |
| ½ cup gravy | 2 |
| 1 cup steamed broccoli | 3.7 |
| 1 cup low-fat milk | 9 |
| 1 medium apple | 0.5 |
| 1 slice whole-wheat bread w/soft tub margarine | 2.7 |

### TOTAL PROTEIN FOR DAY: 125 GRAMS

## MENU #3: HIGH-PROTEIN, LOW-CARBOHYDRATE

| FOOD | PROTEIN (GRAMS) |
|---|---|
| 1 whole-wheat tortilla wrap | 3 |
| 2 scrambled eggs | 12.5 |
| 2 servings turkey bacon | 4.5 |
| 1 cup fresh cantaloupe | 1.5 |
| 1 cup nonfat cottage cheese | 26 |
| 1/3 cup nuts | 5 |
| 1 (4-oz.) grilled chicken breast | 35 |
| 2 cups green salad w/fat-free dressing | 2.3 |
| 1 protein shake | 24 |
| 5 oz. roast beef | 41 |
| 6 spears steamed asparagus | 2 |
| 1 cup low-fat milk | 9 |
| 1 cup fresh strawberries | 1 |
| 1 protein bar | 21 |

### TOTAL PROTEIN FOR DAY:   188 GRAMS

*Source: (for all three menus): USDA Agricultural Research Service Nutrient Database for Standard Research, Release 17.*

## How Many Servings Per Day?

You really need no more than two or three servings of meat or other protein-rich food sources each day. Keep in mind that the commonly served portion size in restaurants is 5 to 7 ounces (and sometimes a lot more)—a portion so big that it really equals two servings of meat. Remember, portions always look bigger on paper than they actually are in real life, so think small. One serving in this group equals:

- Three ounces of meat, poultry, or seafood (about the size and thickness of a deck of cards).
- One egg or two egg whites.
- A fourth of a cup of nuts.
- A fourth of a cup of seeds (like sunflower or pumpkin).

- Half a cup of beans or lentils.

- Two tablespoons peanut butter.

- Half a cup of tofu.

- Half a can of light tuna in water. (Canned albacore tuna can be high in mercury, so don't make this part of your everyday diet.)

Here are some helpful hints for navigating the meat market . . . healthfully:

- Buy lean ground beef or ground turkey *breast* (ground turkey *meat* often has dark meat and skin and therefore a higher fat content).

- Buy "select" or "choice" grades of beef; they have the least marbled fat (streaks of fat between the muscle that cannot be trimmed away). Beef graded "prime" is not only more costly but higher in fat. (Yes, I know this is what makes that prime rib so juicy and tender.) So save these grades of meat for special occasions.

- For beef, look for cuts that have "round" or "loin" in the name, as they are the leanest cuts. Surprisingly, sirloin steak is one of the leanest cuts of meat you can order in a restaurant (order a small portion, of course).

- When shopping for pork, look for the leaner tenderloin or roast cuts.

- For poultry, stick to white meat instead of dark and remove the skin before eating.

- For lamb, choose roasts, chops, or legs for the leanest cuts of meat.

- Buy seafood frozen or fresh but skip the breading and frying.

- Buy albacore or chunk light tuna *in water* instead of oil.

- Buy lean ham or Canadian bacon instead of bacon.

- When shopping for finfish, go for flounder, haddock, salmon, farmed trout, or catfish. Try to avoid swordfish, shark, king mackerel, and fresh tuna, as they can be high in the neurotoxin mercury. (Usually the larger fish are the ones highest in mercury.) Women of childbearing age and children shouldn't eat any seafood that is high in mercury; instead, they can have up to 12 ounces per week (about two servings) of fish lower in mercury (shrimp, canned light tuna, salmon, pollock, farmed catfish, or trout).

- Buy raw or dry-roasted unsalted nuts.

- Buy natural peanut butter that is free of hydrogenation.

- Choose wild or organic salmon to reduce your exposure to harmful chemicals (like dioxins and PCBs) found in some types of farmed salmon.

- Roast, broil, grill, or stir-fry meat instead of frying.

- Try a new dish with tofu, which works great in stir-fry and other vegetarian dishes. You can even buy flavored and precooked tofu.

- Stick to lean, deli-sliced turkey breast, ham, or chicken instead of buying high-sodium, sometimes fatty luncheon meats.

- Trim away all visible fat on meat and poultry.

- Drain visible fat after cooking, especially with ground beef. You can even rinse ground beef with hot water to help remove some fat.

- Brown your meat with nonstick cooking spray instead of butter, oil, or lard.

- Use marinades or fresh herbs to give meat flavor instead of adding salt or fat.

- Use two egg whites rather than one whole egg in omelets or recipes, or try a cholesterol-free egg substitute.

- Keep canned beans on hand to throw into any casserole, stew, or main dish. Or wrap up beans in a warm tortilla with some zesty salsa.

- Be sure to cook meat until the juices run clear and fish until it flakes easily with a fork.

- Avoid eating charred or blackened meats. When cooking meat with a charcoal grill, move the coals to one side so the fat drippings from the meat don't drop directly onto the coals. Charring meat may lead to the development of cancer-causing chemicals during cooking. It is better to cook meat thoroughly on a gas grill at a lower temperature.

- Try to save hot dogs, bologna, sausages, and other mixed and processed meats for special occasions only. This guideline also includes pizza and taco meat from fast-food restaurants.

## What If I Am a Vegetarian?

You don't have to eat meat to enjoy a nutritionally balanced diet. A vegetarian lifestyle can offer a plethora of variety and flavor. With a little planning, vegetarianism is an absolutely healthy way to live. Just remember these simple guidelines:

1. Eat fruits, vegetables, and whole grains at every meal. Try to eat at least one serving of legumes per day. Milk, cheese, or yogurt may be consumed one to three times per day.
2. Eat nuts, seeds, vegetable oils, soy milk, or eggs at least daily.
3. Eat sweets and treats sparingly.
4. Snack on whole grains, fruits, or vegetables between meals.

For strict vegetarians, or vegans (those who do not eat meat, poultry, fish, eggs, or dairy foods), it is important to eat fortified foods. A vegan diet can be low in vitamin D, calcium, iron, zinc, and vitamin B12 (which is found only in animal foods). To get more of these nutrients:

- Eat cereals or margarine spreads that are fortified with vitamin D. Or enjoy ten minutes in the sunlight (without sunscreen, or maybe just your hands or feet) each day, as your body can manufacture vitamin D from sunlight.
- Eat plenty of leafy greens, broccoli, legumes, and tofu for calcium. Try drinking calcium-fortified orange juice.
- Eat beans, peas, leafy greens, prune juice, dried fruit, or fortified breads and cereals for iron.

- Eat fortified cereals, canned beans, wheat germ, wheat bran, and plenty of whole grains for zinc.

- Eat fortified cereals or B12-fortified soy products for vitamin B12.

- Consider a nutritional supplement that contains 100 percent or less of the RDA for vitamin D, calcium, iron, zinc, and vitamin B12.

## Get Adequate Calcium

Our bodies contain more calcium than any other mineral, and 99 percent of it is in our bones and teeth! The average American consumes about 860 milligrams of calcium per day, which is not enough. Depending on age, we should be getting 1,000 to 1,300 milligrams per day.[18] Calcium plays a vital role in metabolism, muscle contraction, blood clotting, regulation of the heartbeat, and nervous-system functions. If that's not good enough, calcium also plays another major role in the body: building strong bones. All of us, young and old, need strong bones, so all of us, young and old, need to make sure we get enough calcium. If calcium intake is too low, we put ourselves at risk for osteoporosis. Osteoporosis means "porous bones" and is the result of genetic, lifestyle, dietary, hormonal, or age-related factors. However, osteoporosis is much more than just weak bones; it can lead to life-altering problems (loss of independence and mobility) that are enormously expensive and physically and emotionally painful. An estimated 10 million Americans have bones weak enough to be diagnosed with osteoporosis (8 million are women). Sadly, another 34 million have bones so weak that they are at risk for fractures. To put this into perspective, one in two women will suffer from an osteoporosis-related fracture in her lifetime.[19] Too many people shrug osteoporosis off as a disease that affects only "old" people, yet the disease actually starts developing at a young age. That means the opportunities to prevent osteoporosis occur much earlier in life than we usually think—like during adolescence. Your bones are actually living tissue—continually in a state of change—sometimes removing calcium for necessary functions (like muscle contractions and heartbeat) and sometimes depositing calcium back into the bone. That is why you must have a consistent supply of calcium to the body. If you are not "depositing" some calcium every day, then you start to lose more calcium than you deposit, leading to a negative calcium balance and poor bone health. Up until the mid-thirties, your body is very efficient at depositing more bone than it removes. However as a natural result of aging, your body starts to lose and/or remove more bone than it is able to deposit. That is why it is so crucial in younger years to get adequate calcium in the diet. Vitamin D also plays a major role in bone health. Vitamin D helps your body to absorb and deposit calcium in your bones and teeth.

There are many risk factors for osteoporosis that you cannot control (like being a woman, being older). However, there are still several factors that you *can* control.

1. Get adequate calcium and vitamin D.
2. Get enough physical activity.
3. Avoid alcohol, smoking, and excessive caffeine (300 milligrams a day or more, which is six [12-ounce] caffeinated drinks per day).

Milk, yogurt, cheese, and even ice cream, along with leafy greens, soybeans, and tofu are all good sources of calcium. Dairy products are a good source of many nutrients. However, their most famous contribution to the human diet is calcium.

## How Much Calcium Do I Need Per Day?

How much calcium you need per day depends on your age:

Since none of us has the time to count up how many milligrams of calcium we eat every day, use this simple rule of thumb: Eat

| AGE | CALCIUM NEEDS PER DAY |
|---|---|
| 9–18 years of age | 1,300 mg per day |
| 19–50 years of age | 1,000 mg per day |
| Over age 50 | 1,200 mg per day |

Source: National Academy of Sciences

at least three servings of calcium-rich food every day. Most calcium-rich foods provide about 300 milligrams per serving. Simply getting three servings will bump you up to about 900 milligrams, and most people consume at least 200 milligrams of calcium per day from other food sources. One serving equals:

- One cup milk, calcium-fortified juice, or soy milk.
- One cup low-fat yogurt.
- One and a half ounce cheese.
- One cup cooked collard greens.

Remember, a single portion is likely smaller than you think. The drinking glasses in my home easily hold 12 fluid ounces, so by enjoying two tall glasses of cold milk each day, I can easily meet my calcium needs.

Calcium doesn't work alone in the body. Magnesium, zinc, fluoride, vitamin D, and likely even vitamin K are all important "assistants" in healthy bone development and maintenance. However, a simple multivitamin mineral supplement with 100 percent of the RDA (no need for more) or a well-balanced diet will provide you with sufficient amounts of these nutrients.

As with most vitamins and minerals, consuming too much calcuim can be toxic. Don't load up on calcium supplements (or any supplements, for that matter) without first consulting your physician. The government's "Tolerable Upper Daily Limit" is set at 2,500 milligrams per day, meaning you shouldn't consume more than 2,500 milligrams of calcium per day.

## Calcium Supplements

- Not all calcium supplements are the same. Read the label.
- Take calcium as a *supplement* to your diet. Tums were never intended to replace calcium from food.

- Try to take supplements with meals and no more than 500 milligrams at a time. But if you don't have the time to take two separate doses, one big dose is better than none at all.
- Drink plenty of fluids with calcium supplements. Milk is a great fluid to wash down your supplement with.

## Helpful Tips

- For snacks, enjoy calcium-rich yogurt, milk, low-fat cheese, or calcium-fortified orange juice or frozen yogurt.
- If you don't like milk, try soy or flavored milks. Or drink milk warm with a little honey or flavoring.
- Eat more dark leafy greens for calcium. Turnip or mustard greens, okra, kale, broccoli, and bok choy are all good vegetable sources of calcium.
- Give tofu a try. It goes great in stir-fry and other dishes. Read the label, as the amount of calcium in tofu can vary.
- Read the label. Many foods, such as cereals and breads, are fortified with calcium.
- If milk gives you bloating, gas, or cramping, you may be lactose intolerant. However, check with your physician before self-diagnosing this condition. If you are lactose intolerant, try drinking lactose-free milk and other less-aggravating dairy foods. You can also try using lactose tablets. Cheese, cottage cheese, and even yogurt are sometimes better tolerated than milk or ice cream.

# Calcium Content in Dairy Foods

| FOOD | PORTION | CALCIUM (in milligrams) | CALORIES |
|---|---|---|---|
| **Milk** | | | |
| 2% | 8 ounce | 285 | 122 |
| 1% | 8 ounce | 290 | 102 |
| Skim | 8 ounce | 306 | 83 |
| Chocolate | 8 ounce | 280 | 208 |
| | | | |
| **Cheese** | | | |
| Muenster | 1.5 ounce | 305 | 156 |
| Cheddar | 1.5 ounce | 307 | 171 |
| Provolone | 1.5 ounce | 321 | 150 |
| Swiss | 1.5 ounce | 336 | 162 |
| Kraft Single | 2 slices | 300 | 62 |
| | | | |
| **Yogurt** | | | |
| Light | 8 ounce | 216 | 125 |
| Whole | 8 ounce | 296 | 149 |
| Low-fat | 8 ounce | 284 | 218 |
| Nonfat–Fruit Variety | 8 ounce | 372 | 230 |
| Custard | 8 ounce | 308 | 258 |
| | | | |
| **Soy** | | | |
| Soybean Curd | 1 ounce | 30 | 22 |
| Soy Milk | 8 ounce | 93 | 127 |
| | | | |
| **Eggs** | | | |
| Egg—Fresh | 1 large | 26 | 74 |
| Scrambled | 1 large | 43 | 101 |

*Source: USDA Agricultrical Research Service Nutrient Database for Standard Reference, Release 17.*

## Calcium Content in Dairy Foods continued...

| FOOD | PORTION | CALCIUM (in milligrams) | CALORIES |
|---|---|---|---|
| Ice-Cream | | | |
| Vanilla | 1/2 cup | 92 | 145 |
| Fat Free | 1/2 cup | 83 | 93 |
| Light | 1/2 cup | 122 | 125 |
| Light–Soft Serve | 1/2 cup | 138 | 111 |
| Frozen Yogurt | 1/2 cup | 103 | 117 |

Source: *USDA Agriculturial Research Service Nutrient Database for Standard Reference, Release 17.*

# Eating on the Run

Quick! Which would you choose on a hectic morning where the alarm didn't go off, the dog ate the kids' homework, the car keys turned up missing, and now you have only ten seconds to find something for breakfast to get you through a rough morning?

1. Fast food egg and sausage muffin.
2. Bakery cinnamon roll.
3. Yogurt and banana (from a gas station).
4. Bakery bagel with cream cheese.
5. Drive-through pancakes with margarine and syrup.

For the lowest number of calories (some foods are higher in sodium or fat than others, even if the calories are lower), the fast food egg and sausage muffin, at 290 calories, is your best bet. Surprised? Frankly, so was I. For good health, the yogurt and banana is an excellent option because of the fiber, protein, calcium, and lower fat content. But many of us, in a frenzy like this, are looking for a "drive-through" quick-fix.

Here are the choices again with calories per serving exposed:

1. Fast food egg and sausage muffin: 290 calories.

2. Bakery cinnamon roll: 700–1,300 calories.

3. Yogurt and banana: 300–350 calories.

4. Bakery bagel with cream cheese: 430 calories.

5. Pancakes from drive-through: 600 calories.

Telling someone to "eat healthy" in the unpredictable world of fast-food is an uphill battle; it is just too hard to know what you're eating when you don't have the luxury of seeing the food prepared and don't have a food label to look at or the time to care (and when you can wolf down an entire meal in a matter of minutes).

This problem is compounded by the fact that we dine away from home quite frequently. Eating meals away from home used to be an "occasional" indulgence. However, in today's life in the fast lane, many of us rely on food away from home just to get through the day. Eating out can be healthful, halfway decent, or downright artery-clogging and unhealthy. Most entrees are served in portions that are too large and pack too many calories, too much fat, and too much sodium.

If you're one of the lucky ones, and you eat out only one to two times per week or less, you can probably enjoy your restaurant food without much ado. However, if you eat food away from home more than two times per week, you need to make it a point to order wisely—for your health. Here are several tips (plenty of them!) to help you learn how. Keep in mind that when I recommend skipping certain items, it isn't just because the food has *slightly* more calories, fat, or sodium. I usually tell you to skip something for good reason.

## Restaurant Tips

My job requires occasional travel. On one trip, I sat down hoping to enjoy a quiet dinner and catch up on some reading. What I got was much more fun. I was attending a dietitian convention, and it didn't take long to realize that fellow nutritionists and health nuts surrounded me. As I sat quietly and tried to enjoy a dinner of very dry salmon and withered carrots, I couldn't help but listen to the commotion. I came in too late to catch the saga at the table next to me as the people ordered their dinner, but I was right there—within earshot—when their food came. They were not happy. "I ordered the club sandwich dry, with no mayo or mustard," said one woman. "I ordered the club sandwich with no bacon and only mustard," said another. "I wanted a side salad with vinegar, not ranch, instead of fries," snapped another. One man sent his steak back because it was too raw. "This is simply not cooked well enough," he said, patronizing the poor waitress. When the waitress brought the steak back to the table, it was, of course, "overcooked." "Yikes! No wonder nobody likes to go out to eat with a dietitian," I thought. I am sure this was just a freak thing—dietitians are very cool people! But my point is that restaurants will accommodate your requests; they understand that we are simply concerned about our health. And if they can handle a room full of dietitians, they can certainly handle a healthy-request table here and there. And maybe, just maybe, restaurants will start to serve healthier dishes if we make it known that we want them (this seems to be happening as I write this). You should be patient and understanding, though, as most restaurants do make honest attempts to accommodate special requests.

Here are more restaurant tips:

- Skip appetizers. If you must indulge, try chips and salsa, lettuce wraps, or seafood cocktail. You might also try ordering an appetizer for your main course. (An appetizer of cheese fries with ranch dressing can pack 3,000 calories and 217 grams of fat [91 of them saturated and trans fat[20]]—more than four times the amount of *bad* fat you should have in one day). How smooth and creamy would 18 tablespoons—yes, over a full cup—of solid vegetable shortening taste going down?

- Avoid drinking your calories. Restaurant food is already high enough in calories. The last thing you need is an additional 250 to 650 calories in a sugary beverage.

- Order foods that have been grilled, roasted, baked, broiled, or stir-fried.

- Avoid menu items that use words like "fried," "breaded," "batter-dipped," "buttery," "creamed," "sautéed," "rich," or "crispy."
- Order gravy, salad dressing, and rich sauces (such as béarnaise) on the side.
- Think simple. Often ordering a grilled piece of fish or chicken and a dinner salad is one of your best options.
- Don't clean your plate. Restaurant portions tend to be large (except in expensive, five-star restaurants). Plan on taking half of your food home for later. Or try splitting an entrée with a friend.
- Don't overdo it at the salad bar. The salad bar is a healthful option at almost any restaurant. However, when you start adding eggs, cheese, nuts, beans, meats, and full-fat salad dressing, things start to add up—fast! Check this out:

| | |
|---|---|
| 2 cups leafy greens | 20 calories |
| 4 slices cucumber | 6 calories |
| 1/4 cup grated carrots | 12 calories |
| 1/4 cup green peas | 31 calories |
| 4 cherry tomatoes | 12 calories |
| 1 T. sunflower seed kernels | 47 calories |
| 2 T. fat-free dressing | 48 calories |
| Total | 176 calories |

*Now, take off the fat-free dressing and add all of this:*

| | |
|---|---|
| 1/4 cup shredded cheese | 100 calories |
| 5 olives | 42 calories |
| 1/4 cup chopped boiled eggs | 53 calories |
| 1 oz. lean turkey | 27 calories |
| 2 T. kidney beans | 28 calories |
| 2 T. croutons | 15 calories |
| 1/4 cup regular salad dressing | 300 calories |
| New Total | 693 calories |

*Source: USDA Agricultural Research Service Nutrient Database for Standard Reference, Release 17.*

Even though many of these things are healthful, it is wiser to load up on the vegetables or fruits at the salad bar. If you go with full-fat salad dressing, try to choose only one other topping that is calorie dense (beans, eggs, meat, cheese, olives, nuts, or seeds). If you stick to fat-free dressing, you can enjoy three or four of those calorie-dense toppings.

For a detailed list of restaurant tips for ethnic foods, see the appendix.

## Eating Sensibly: A Summary

Who knew there was so much meaning behind the words "eat sensibly"? Nutrition is a tricky, confusing, and ever-changing world, yet it affects our lives and our precious health at fundamental levels every day. With a plentiful food supply, declining health, and never-ending nutrition information at your fingertips, your health is worth the time it takes to learn accurate and helpful nutrition information. In other words, in today's society, good health is not just going to drop into your lap—you have to fight for it!

Here is a quick review of each of the recommendations I gave to help you eat a healthful yet realistic diet:

1. Read the food label.
2. Shrink serving sizes.
3. Focus on plant-based foods (whole grains, fruits, vegetables, legumes, nuts, seeds) and fiber for health and weight management.
4. Consume healthy fats in moderation (monounsaturated fats from canola, olive oil, nuts, and avocados, and Omega-3 fats from fish, flaxseed, or canola oil).
5. Use lean meats and other protein-rich foods in moderation.
6. Get adequate calcium from food.
7. Eat sensibly, even when you are on the run.

This may seem like a lot of information to focus on all at once, so don't hesitate to pick one thing at a time to work on. Changing our eating habits is downright hard. But any change in the right direction is good, so start with small goals and go for it. Always remember: balance, variety, and moderation are the keys to good health.

All of these recommendations are incorporated into the meal plan at the back of this book. The meal plan includes delicious recipes, easy-to-prepare meals, and quick but healthy snack options, all of which stick to the guidelines I've presented. There are even a few snacks that are not so healthy (like chocolate!) but can still be a realistic part of our ever-stressful, project-packed lives. With a little balance and discipline, being "too busy" to eat healthy is no longer a good excuse.

## Notes

1. Dave Barry (used by permission).

2. J. Putnam, J. Allshouse, and L. Scott Kantor, "U.S. Per Capita Food Supply Trends: More Calories, Refined Carbohydrates, and Fats," *Food Review,* vol. 25, no. 3 (USDA Economic Research Service, 2002).

3. *Journal of Discourses,* 26 vols. (London: Latter-day Saints' Book Depot, 1854–86), 13:153–54.

4. *Doctrine and Covenants Student Manual* (Salt Lake City: The Church of Jesus Christ of Latter-day Saints, 1981), 206–11.

5. S. P. Murphy and R. K. Johnson, "The Scientific Basis of Recent U.S. Guidance on Sugars Intake," *American Journal of Clinical Nutrition,* 2003; 78(supplement):827s–833s.

6. *Behavioral Risk Factor Surveillance Survey* (Nationwide 2003 Prevalence Data), http://apps.nccd.cdc.gov/brfss/display.asp?cat=FV&yr=2003&qkey=4415&state=US.

7. J. S. Carson, F. M. Burke, and L. A. Hark, eds., *Cardiovascular Nutrition—Disease Management and Prevention* (The American Dietetic Association, 2004).

8. C. Taylor, *Qualified Health Claims: Letter of Enforcement Discretion—Nuts and Coronary Heart Disease,* http://vm.cfsan.fda.gov/~dms/qhcnuts2.html.

9. J. S. Carson, F. M. Burke, and L. A. Hark, eds., *Cardiovascular Nutrition—Disease Management and Prevention* (The American Dietetic Association, 2004), 230.

10. Kathleen L. Mahon and Sylvia Escott-Stump, *Krause's Food, Nutrition, and Diet Therapy,* 9th ed. (Philadelphia: W. B. Saunders, 1996).

11. N. C. Howarth, E. Saltzman, and S. B. Roberts, "Dietary Fiber and Weight Regulation," *Nutrition Reviews,* 2001; 59(5):129–39.

12. Roberta L. Duyff, *The American Dietetic Association's Complete Food and Nutrition Guide* (Chronimed Publishing, 1998), 149.

13. Kathleen L. Mahon and Sylvia Escott-Stump, *Krause's Food, Nutrition, and Diet Therapy,* 9th ed. (Philadelphia: W. B. Saunders, 1996), 59.

14. *Intake of Calories and Selected Nutrients for the United States Population, 1999–2000.* U.S. Department of Health and Human Services, Centers for Disease Control, National Center for Health Statistics.

15. D. B. Allison, S. K. Egan, L. M. Barraj, C. Caughman, M. Infante, and J. T. Heimbach, "Estimated Intakes of Trans Fatty and Other Fatty Acids in the U.S. Population," *Journal of the American Dietetic Association,* 1999:99; 2:166–69.

16. D. B. Allison, S. K. Egan, L. M. Barraj, C. Caughman, M. Infante, and J. T. Heimbach, "Estimated Intakes of Trans Fatty and Other Fatty Acids in the U.S. Population," *Journal of the American Dietetic Association,* 1999; 99(2):166–69.

17. P. Trumbo, S. Schlicker, A. Yates, and M. Poos, "Dietary Reference Intakes for Energy, Carbohydrate, Fiber, Fat, Fatty Acids, Cholesterol, Protein and Amino Acids." *Journal of the American Dietetic Association,* 2002; 102(11):1621–25.

18. J. Wright, C. Wang, J. Kennedy-Stephenson, and R. B. Ervin, "Dietary Intake of Ten Key Nutrients for Public Health, United States: 1999–2000," *Advance Data from Vital Health and Statistics,* no. 334 (Centers for Disease Control and Prevention).

19. National Institutes of Health website: Osteo.org/newfile.asp?doc=fast&doctitle=fast+facts+on+osteoporosis&doctype=HTML+fact+sheet.

20. M. F. Jacobson and J. G. Hurley, *Restaurant Confidential* (New York: Workman Publishing, 2002).

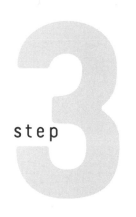

# Get Moving

**step 3**

**KEY POINTS:**

Understanding the Benefits of Exercise | What Kind of Exercise Should I Do? | The How, When, and What of Aerobic Exercise | The How, When, and What of Strength Training | Balancing Food Intake and Exercise

## Understanding the Benefits of Exercise

"In the bottle before you is a pill, a marvel of modern medicine that will regulate gene transcription throughout your body, helping you prevent heart disease, stroke, diabetes, obesity, and twelve kinds of cancer—plus gallstones and diverticulitis. Expect the pill to improve your strength and balance as well as your blood-lipid profile. Your bones will become stronger. You'll grow new capillaries in your heart, your skeletal muscle, and your brain, improving blood flow and the delivery of oxygen and nutrients. Your attention span will increase. If you have arthritis, your symptoms will improve. The pill will help you regulate your appetite, and you'll probably find you prefer healthier foods. You'll feel better—younger, even—and will test younger according to a variety of physiological measures. Your blood volume will increase, and you'll burn fats better. Even your immune system will be stimulated. There's just one catch: There's no such pill. The prescription is exercise."[1]

This statement is not just an uplifting quotation that attempts to get you to exercise. Exercise really does reduce the risk of many diseases that plague us and our loved ones. And without a doubt, exercise is a powerful promoter of good health. How many of us would drop

[ 81 ]

everything to buy one of those pills right now? How many of us would park far, far away and walk for fifteen minutes, in each direction, to get to the "research lab" and pick up one of those revolutionary pills? The point is that, on average, most people will trust a pill to give them a desired result. Many of us trust in medications to control our blood pressure, our cholesterol, and even to regulate the delicate beating of our hearts. Sometimes life or death situations are left in the hands of a simple pill. But how many of us really trust in exercise enough to devote a trivial thirty minutes out of our busy day to doing it? "Exercise is often overlooked. . . . Exercise can change virtually every tissue in the body, but because it works by many different pathways—metabolic, hormonal, neurological, and mechanical—understanding why and how it works, in an integrated way, is not easy."[2]

An editorial in the *New England Journal of Medicine* reviewed several studies relating to the power of exercise in reducing the risk of death, and guess what the bottom line was? "Greater fitness results in longer survival."[3] Even in the 1800s, President Brigham Young knew the value of exercise as he candidly said, "Many persons are so constituted, that if you put them in a parlor, keep a good fire for them, furnish them tea, cake, sweet meats, etc., and nurse them tenderly, soaking their feet, and putting them to bed, they will die in a short time; but throw them into snow banks, and they will live a great many years."[4]

Aside from the scientific evidence corroborating the vital need for physical activity, we also know that there are spiritual reasons for engaging in healthful activity patterns. The Lord has always shown concern for our physical health. Our bodies are so important that the Lord calls them "temples of God" and the dwelling place for our precious spirits (see 1 Corinthians 3:16–17).

I remember going through a time in which I was stressed out to the max. Work was hectic. I was spending all day and many a night at my computer, and my skin felt as if it were growing attached to my office chair. I wasn't eating healthy or feeding my family healthy, and I was missing all of my workouts. One day after working long hours, I was sitting at my kitchen table trying to finish up my work when my four-year-old daughter began to ask me "why" questions (like "Why is the sky blue?" and "Why do we eat cows?"). After about the sixteenth question and the sixteenth angry answer, my four-year-old finally stopped in her tracks and studied me. With her hands on her hips and a stern glare she said, "Are you my mother?" It took about one second for me to realize I had completely lost touch with my priorities. But later I realized something else: Exercise helps me control my mood. Now, this is only the science of Melanie Douglass, but I believe, with every inch of my living soul, that exercise is a powerful and reliable way to lift your spirits and ward off depression, anxiety, or mood swings. Of course, I am not saying you will never again yell at your children. I simply believe that in addition to all of the miracle benefits of exercise, regular physical activity helps you be a happier person.

The media seems to blast us every day with more doomsday statistics about how inactive we are. However, some of this criticism is well deserved. Sixty-eight percent of Americans fail to meet even the minimum government recommendation for thirty minutes of moderate-intensity exercise on most days of the week.[5] Think about all of the wonderful luxuries we enjoy: television, cars, elevators, escalators, remote controls, and washing machines. Those things are obvious, but what about the things that are absolutely unnecessary, like DVD players that play six DVDs? (Yes, that's a good twelve hours attached to the couch.) What about drive-throughs? Do we really not have time to get out of the car and walk a few steps to pick up a 1,000-calorie meal? Even things like riding lawn mowers, leaf blowers, autopilot vacuums, and the ability to run your life with a computer, a phone, and a chair are contributing to this ever-growing problem. Bit by bit, all of the missed opportunities to burn a calorie here and there are adding up, and our health is paying the price for it. The bottom line is simple: Exercise is no longer something we do just to lose a few pounds; exercise is something we *must* make time for. It is absolutely necessary to maintain good health.

So now we know why we should exercise, but actually doing it can be hard. Believe me, I understand. I have a four-year-old, a three-year-old, and a three-month-old. (Enough said, right?) Often, when I start a workout in my home, I make it about ten minutes before someone needs a drink, someone needs to go potty, the phone rings, dinner starts to burn, and yes, the entire house is on the verge of falling apart—all because Mom wanted just a few minutes to herself! There seems to be no shortage of excuses for not exercising: You're embarrassed to be seen in workout clothes, or to sweat next to complete strangers at the gym. You have kids that you can't leave alone. It's too cold outside, too hot, or too wet. You haven't prepared your church lesson yet, and it's time to make dinner, and—oh, yeah—American Idol is on.

We all have other things to do, but we get only one shot with this precious body, and it deserves a little bit of time each day. After all, if we don't take care of ourselves, what will we have to give our family and friends? So get out that list of excuses and get ready to cross off each and every one. I am about to clear up the confusion regarding the what, when, and how of exercise—and give some great tips for anybody, anywhere, at any time to *get moving*.

## What Kind of Exercise Should I Do?

There are two main types of exercise, both of which have important roles in achieving and maintaining good health. The first one is aerobic exercise (also known as cardiorespiratory training), and the second one is strength (or resistance) training. Both are extremely beneficial to the body, and one is not necessarily more important than the other. Aerobic exercise strengthens your heart and lungs through activities that are rhythmic and continuous. Strength training involves using some form of resistance: hand weights, resistance tubing, machines, or even gravity for shorter, more intense periods of time, in order to improve muscular strength and power. We'll discuss strength training in greater detail later in the chapter. And at the end of the book, I'll explain how to put together a complete workout program that fits both your schedule and your budget.

## Aerobic Exercise

*What is aerobic exercise?* Aerobic exercise simply means that your body is using and metabolizing oxygen to produce energy for sustained periods of activity. Good examples of aerobic activity are walking, jogging, biking, swimming, aerobics, stair-climbing, and rowing. Treadmills offer an unbeatable workout, thanks to the consistent drive of a smooth motor. Elliptical trainers and recumbent bikes also offer a great workout for all fitness levels. Regular aerobic exercise helps your heart pump more blood with each beat and decreases the amount of work your heart has to do to distribute oxygen and nutrients throughout your body. Aerobic exercise burns calories, promotes a healthy metabolism, and tones your body. In my experience as a personal trainer, I have also seen aerobic exercise boost energy levels, decrease feelings of anxiety and depression, and help people sleep better.

## How Many Times Per Week Do I Need Aerobic Exercise?

*The Dietary Guidelines for Americans 2005,* put out by the U.S. Department of Health and Human Services and the U.S. Department of Agriculture in agreement with the U.S. Surgeon General, recommends that Americans get moderate physical activity on most days of the week.[6] Ideally, this translates to four to six days per week. For some of us, that may sound completely unrealistic. However, we all have to start somewhere, and taking the first step is never easy, but it is always rewarding. If you currently exercise one day per week, try working out two days per week. If you currently exercise three days per week, try upping it to four days, and so forth. It is perfectly okay to set small, realistic, and achievable goals in order to work toward the goal of "most days of the week." Every bout of exercise counts. Stanford's William Haskell, in an interview with the Center for Science in the Public Interest's Bonnie Leibman, said this: "Take a 50-year-old man who is somewhat overweight and typically has moderately elevated blood sugar, triglycerides, or blood pressure, . . . a single bout of exercise of moderate intensity—like 30 to 40 minutes of brisk walking—will lower those numbers."[7]

## How Long Do My Aerobic Workouts Need to Last?

The good news is that you don't need to run a marathon. The new *Dietary Guidelines for Americans* gives the following recommendations regarding exercise duration:

- Thirty minutes of moderate intensity activity on most days of the week to reduce the risk of chronic disease in adulthood.

- Sixty minutes of moderate intensity activity on most days of the week to manage body weight and prevent gradual, unhealthy body weight gain in adulthood.

- Sixty to ninety minutes of moderate intensity activity on most days of the week to sustain weight loss in adulthood.[8]

Although it's great if you can work out consistently for thirty to sixty minutes at a time, your efforts are still worthwhile and beneficial even if you break up your exercise throughout the day. We all used to be under the assumption that if you couldn't exercise for at least thirty minutes, it wasn't worth the effort. The argument was that if you wanted to "burn fat" and not "sugar" then you had to work out for a longer period of time. We know that the most efficient fat-burning stage of our workout does occur after activity has been sustained for a longer period of time, but we also know that a calorie is a calorie. The bottom line is that we need to *burn calories*, and whether those calories come from fat stores or glucose (carbohydrate) stores is irrelevant. Every bout, whether it lasts two minutes, ten minutes, or sixty minutes, burns calories. Consider this: If you were to get up and do twenty-five jumping jacks right now, do you think your body would refuse to burn a single calorie, just because you didn't maintain the activity for twenty minutes? Absolutely not! Every muscle action requires energy, and therefore, every muscle action burns calories.

## How Intense Do My Workouts Need to Be?

No pain, no gain—right? Actually, no. This is a common myth in the exercise world. Current research tells us that moderate-intensity exercise is the most beneficial for weight management, reduced risk of disease, and overall good health. Moderate intensity can mean different things to different people. For an elderly person, it may mean walking at two miles per hour, whereas a forty-year-old may walk at four miles per hour. In general, you should feel challenged but comfortable during your workouts. That means you should be able to speak or carry on a light conversation, but you should not be able to chat away effortlessly. If you can sing the national anthem while you work out, it is probably time to take the intensity up a notch. Another tool to measure intensity is the Borg Rating of Perceived Exertion (RPE) scale.[9] This is a tool in which you assign a number to how you feel. The scale looks like this:

| | |
|---|---|
| **6** | No exertion at all |
| **7–8** | Extremely light (7.5) |
| **9** | Very Light |
| **10** | |
| **11** | Light |
| **12** | |
| **13** | Somewhat hard |
| **14** | |
| **15** | Hard (heavy) |
| **16** | |
| **17** | Very Hard |
| **18** | |
| **19** | Extremely Hard |
| **20** | Maximal Exertion |

| | |
|---|---|
| **9** | corresponds to "very light" exercise. For a healthy person, it is like walking slowly at his or her own pace for some minutes |
| **13** | on the scale is "somewhat hard" exercise, but it still feels OK to continue. |
| **17** | "very hard" is very strenuous. A healthy person can still go on, but he or she really has to push him- or herself. It feels very heavy, and the person is very tired. |
| **19** | on the scale is an extremely strenuous exercise level. For most people this is the most strenuous exercise they have ever experienced. |

*Borg RPE scale*
*© Gunnar Borg, 1970, 1985, 1994, 1998*

The Borg Scale is a great tool. For most people, activity performed at a rating of 12 to 14 generally suggests that activity is being performed at a "moderate" intensity level.

Another tool to help you gauge workout intensity is "target heart rate." While working out, we want to challenge the heart and lungs but not overstress them. Target heart rate is the optimal number of heartbeats per minute at which you work out. Target heart rate is calculated in the following way:

1. Measure your resting heart rate (RHR). The best time for measurement is in the morning, right after you wake up. Take your pulse and count the number of heartbeats in sixty seconds.

2. Calculate your maximum heart rate (MHR). Subtract your age from the number 220. If you are 50, then 220 – 50 = 170, your MHR.

4. Subtract your resting heart rate (RHR) from your maximum heart rate (MHR). If you are 50 years old with a MHR of 170, and your measured RHR is 70, then 170 – 70 = 100.

5. Multiply this number by the target heart rate (THR) percentage. We will use the general recommendation of 60 to 90 percent. So, .60 x 100 = 60 (lower range) and .90 x 100 = 90 (upper range).

6. Add your resting heart rate back to these numbers. For example, 60 + 70 = 130 lower range, 90 + 70 = 160 upper range.

Target heart rate is simply a recommended "range" for your heart rate to stay within while you work out. The general recommendation is to work somewhere between 60 to 90 percent of your maximum heart rate. A heart-rate monitor is a great tool to help you gauge your workout intensity and cardiovascular progress as your body becomes more efficient with exercise.

To translate this information into a real workout, "moderate" intensity may mean walking on a treadmill at three miles per hour. But remember, the whole point of exercise is to build a stronger, healthier, more efficient body. Therefore, as the three-miles-per-hour pace becomes easier, you will have to increase speed or add incline to keep your body challenged. Essentially, when you finally master a certain workout and it is no longer challenging, it is *time to change your routine or make it more difficult.* That doesn't mean your workouts have to be painful, just challenging. In addition, think of how exciting it will be to know that you won't be stuck in the same workout rut for the rest of your life. A new challenge is what motivates the human body to continue down a path. Progression is vital for physical and spiritual growth.

# Strength Training

For many people aerobic activity is a no-brainer—we all know how to walk, ride a bike, or follow a simple home-exercise video. But strength training, for many people, takes on a whole new realm of complexity. It's hard to know which exercises to do, how often to do them, how many of them to do, and how to do them correctly in order to avoid injuries. To implement a maintainable strength-training program into your life, you must first understand the importance of this type of exercise.

## Why Is Strength Training So Important?

The first thing strength training does is increase muscle mass. "Muscle is the absolute centerpiece for being healthy, vital, and independent as we grow older."[10] The most appealing benefit of strength training is that it boosts our metabolism (because of the increased lean body mass and decreased body fat percentage); makes us leaner; improves self-esteem and confidence; reduces back pain by improving the back's strength, flexibility, and endurance; and reduces the risk and severity of osteoporosis, falls, and fractures as we age. Strength training also increases connective tissue strength to improve joint stability and reduce the risk of injury. And whether your goal is to kick a soccer ball with more power or to pick up a bag of groceries, strength training is vital to improve functional strength not only for sports but also for common daily activities. Strength training even contributes to the prevention and management of a variety of chronic medical conditions, such as diabetes, heart disease, and osteoarthritis.[11] On top of all that, strength training makes you look and feel great! There. Enough said. Do we really need any more reasons to pick up a set of hand weights?

## Debunking the Myths of Strength Training

*Myth 1: "Strength training makes women too bulky."* I have met so many women who are terrified of strength training because they are afraid it will build big, bulky muscles. The truth is that for most women, strength training simply means building a strong body from the inside out. In fact, as we've discussed, lean muscle tissue takes up less space than fat tissue, so instead of "bulking up," most women lose inches! Men, however, have more lean muscle tissue from the start, and they therefore have the natural capability to add bulk and size through a moderate-to-heavy strength-training program. This is because men are taller, wider, and have larger body frames and higher levels of testosterone. Because women naturally have less muscle and bone mass, women are at a greater risk for osteoporosis and disability with age, so women need to do strength training just as much as, if not more than, men. Think of strength training as a form of exercise that will keep you healthy, active, independent, strong, and lean for the rest of your life.

*Myth 2: "I'm too old to start a strength-training program."* You are never too old, too young, too out of shape, or too disabled to benefit from a well-designed strength-training program. Children as young as eight years old as well as ninety-eight-year-old nursing-home residents can benefit from age-appropriate strength training. A Tufts University study found that even frail nursing-home residents benefited from strength training. The residents improved their muscle strength, walking speed, and ability to climb stairs in just ten weeks.[12] However, that doesn't mean just anybody can jump into a rigorous strength-training program. Anyone with health conditions or risk factors for disease should definitely consult a physician before beginning a new exercise program. But just because you have to consult a physician doesn't mean you won't benefit from an exercise program. In fact, you are probably the kind of person who will see the greatest benefit. Consulting a health professional may just mean that you need to engage in a supervised, age-appropriate strength-training program. Strength training is vital to our health but sometimes requires professional customization and application because of certain health conditions. So yes, sometimes it will take a small financial investment—a physician's visit, a meeting with a personal trainer, or maybe a consultation with a physical therapist in order to get started. This small financial investment is a minor inconvenience when you think of the heavy cost and emotional suffering associated with the lack of physical activity.

*Myth 3: "Spot training is a more focused option."* Oh, how I wish it were true! How many of us would love to save precious minutes every day and exercise only the one area that needs to lose a few pounds—our arms, our unfortunate spare tire, or even our thighs. Sorry, but the theory of "spot-training" is a myth; the human body doesn't work that way. Here's an example of what I mean: Let's say your abdominal area is a little flabby, so you start to do 100 crunches every night before bed. Eventually, your abdominal muscles become strong and firm. But something is not right—your stomach area still looks loose and flabby. The problem is that your abdominal muscles are actually beneath a layer of subcutaneous fat. Even if you had abs of steel, you would never see them under a layer of excess fat. Only losing weight through a healthy diet and regular exercise can get rid of the unwanted extra fat. And where you lose the fat first is quite unpredictable—it mostly depends on your genes.

*Myth 4: "Walking with light weights on my arms or legs can count as my strength training."* In most instances, the one-, two-, or even three-pound arm or leg weights used during an aerobic exercise such as walking will do you almost no good. The weights are simply not heavy enough to count as strength training. The purpose of strength training is to challenge, or apply stress, to the muscle. This is typically done by using an amount of weight that can be lifted eight to fifteen times in a row. If you can lift a certain amount of weight more than twelve to fifteen times, then it is probably too light to bring you any strength-training benefits.

*Myth 5: "No pain, no gain."* There are two kinds of pain to consider here: pain during exercise and pain after exercise. Neither is necessary to see exercise benefits. During exercise, it is okay to feel muscle fatigue or a "burning" sensation. However, sharp, jarring, grating, popping, or grinding pains are bad. If you ever experience this kind of pain, you need to stop the exercise immediately and consult a physician. In regard to pain after exercise, many people still believe that a workout was too easy if, after exercising, they can still walk, use the bathroom, or sit down in a chair without emitting a few muffled cries of pain. Of course, that isn't true. Occasional soreness is perfectly okay, especially when you are just starting a new workout program. However, painful, activity-limiting soreness on a regular basis is not okay.

*Myth 6: "To burn more calories, lift the weight as fast as you can."* Not only is lifting weights quickly much less effective than lifting them slowly, but lifting too fast can put you at risk for an exercise-induced injury! A slower tempo is safer and more effective; it allows you to focus on your form so you can really feel the contraction on the way up and on the way down. Try something: Place your left hand on your right bicep (the front of your upper arm between the elbow and shoulder joint) and close your eyes. Without any mental or physical effort, let your arm bend at the elbow, and bring your palm toward your shoulder for a bicep curl. Easy, right? Now try it a different way: Mentally focus on your bicep muscle and make it contract and tighten. Next, keep that strong contraction in your bicep and bring your palm up toward the shoulder for another bicep curl. Now, don't lose that contraction. Lower your palm back down and resist the contraction. Finally, after you have gone through the full range of motion for a bicep curl, let your bicep muscle relax. Did you feel a difference? I hope so. Often, when you perform strength-training exercises too fast, you lose that mental focus and the ability to go through the full range of motion. Lifting faster doesn't burn more calories—recruiting more muscle fibers burns more calories. A good rule of thumb is to slowly count two counts up and two counts down. That translates into five to eight seconds per repetition.

## How Do I Get Started with a Strength-Training Program?

Before you get started with a strength-training program, it is important to understand a few terms: *sets, reps* or *repetitions, intensity,* and *rest time.* A *rep* refers to the number of times you repeat an exercise. Ten reps means repeating the same exercise ten times. A *set* is the number of repetitions of an exercise performed in row. *Intensity* refers to how much weight you lift, or how much stress you place on the muscle. Light intensity means that the weight or resistance you use is light enough to allow you to complete 15 to 20 repetitions of an exercise without fatiguing. Light intensity is geared toward beginners and those who wish to build muscular endurance. Medium intensity means the weight or resistance is heavy enough to allow you to complete 10 to 15 repetitions before fatiguing. Medium intensity is where most of us need to be training; it promotes muscular strength and functionality, and it tones and firms the body. Heavy-intensity exercise means the weight or resistance is heavy enough that you can complete only 6 to 10 reps before fatiguing. Heavy intensity is for the more experienced strength trainer and is used mainly for adding bulk, size, strength, and power. The last term to become familiar with is *rest time.* This one is easy and enjoyable. Rest time is simply the amount of time you rest—do nothing but breathe—between sets.

So if I tell you that you need to do three sets of 10 repetitions at a medium intensity and rest for 30 seconds between sets, how does that translate into your next workout? Well, your workout would look something like this:

*Strength Training Program, Day 1*

1. Warm up for 5 to 10 minutes.

2. Exercise 1: Wall squat. Complete 10 repetitions (set 1).

3. Rest 30 seconds.

4. Exercise 1: Wall squat. Complete 10 repetitions (set 2).

5. Rest 30 seconds.

6. Exercise 1: Wall squat. Complete 10 repetitions (set 3).

7. Rest 30 seconds.

8. Exercise 2: Bicep curl. Complete 10 repetitions (set 1).

9. Rest 30 seconds.

10. Continue the cycle.

In this book there is an eight-week strength-training program. The workout is designed for those who own a simple stability ball and resistance band or hand weights. The workout will tell you exactly what exercises to do, how to do them, and in what order to do them for each of the eight weeks of your program. All you have to do is find the time to complete the workouts two to three times per week. One way to save time during your workouts is to try circuit training.

## What Is Circuit Training?

Circuit training is a time- and calorie-efficient method to complete strength-training workouts. Circuit training essentially removes the rest period of your workouts. But because you can't (and shouldn't be able to) do three sets of the same exercise without resting, you instead do one set of *every* exercise and *then* rest. So if I tell you that you need to do three sets of ten repetitions in a circuit, here's what I mean:

*Strength Training Program, Day 1 (Circuit Workout)*

1. Warm up for 5 to 10 minutes.
2. Exercise 1: Wall squat. 10 reps (set 1).
3. Exercise 2: Bent-over row. 10 reps (set 1).
4. Exercise 3: Chest press. 10 reps (set 1).
5. Exercise 4: Shoulder press. 10 reps (set 1).
6. Exercise 5: Biceps curl. 10 reps (set 1).
7. Exercise 6: Triceps pushdown. 10 reps (set 1).
8. Exercise 7: Abdominal curl. 10 reps (set 1).
9. Rest for 1 to 2 minutes.
10. Complete set 2 of all seven exercises.
11. Rest for 1 to 2 minutes.
12. Complete set 3 of all seven exercises.
13. Rest for 1 to 2 minutes.

If you are constantly pressed for time (and who isn't?), then circuit training is a *great* way to get your strength-training workouts done. Circuit training is also an efficient way to work out because you burn calories and enjoy yourself more because of the constant change and quick pace of the workout. In my opinion, the time-saving benefit of circuit training is the way to go; the last thing our excuse-ridden society needs is more excuses not to exercise!

## How Many Times Per Week Do I Need to Do Strength Training?

The American College of Sports Medicine recommends that strength training be done two to three days per week. Although I still stand by my lifelong motto of "Everything you do counts," strength training one day or less per week is not optimal because there is a risk for injury or unnecessary weekly muscle soreness. A good rule of thumb is to allow one day of rest after each strength-training session. So for a total-body workout, three alternating days per week is great. Those who like to strength train on most days of the week can simply do a split routine. For example, Monday and Wednesday would be an upper-body workout, and Tuesday and Thursday would be a lower-body workout. This kind of routine allows you to train on consecutive days without overstressing your muscles.

Remember, this book includes a detailed eight-week strength-training program. The exercise name, how-to, sets, and reps are all outlined for a complete total-body workout.

## Balancing Food Intake and Exercise

It is very hard for me to say this—really, really hard in fact. But here goes: Exercise doesn't burn a lot of calories. However, don't ever forget about all the amazing benefits of exercise, only one of which is weight loss. Exercise helps you ward off disease, builds a strong and healthy body, improves self-esteem, fights depression and anxiety, helps you sleep better, helps you manage stress better, and provides an overall sense of well-being.

The reason I say exercise doesn't burn a lot of calories is that our capability to eat too many calories exceeds (by a long shot) the amount of calories we can realistically burn in a normal workout. Imagine this scenario: Michelle has just started working out after years of being inactive. She goes to the gym after work and jogs at a quick five miles per hour on the treadmill for thirty minutes. She is dripping wet with sweat from her great workout—she just burned 340 calories. Michelle takes a quick shower at the club and then jumps in her car to meet her friends for dinner at the local pasta house. Michelle orders salad with dressing, two breadsticks, and a plate of fettuccini alfredo. Michelle is starving and feels great after her invigorating workout, so she gobbles up every bite of this savory dinner. However, Michelle just ate 2,100 calories! It will take her more than six workouts—

yes, three hours—to burn off that one meal. This scenario isn't exclusive to just sit-down restaurants with friends. You can make a quick stop at a convenience store or fast-food drive-through and eat 500 to 1,000 calories as you wait at a traffic light! So yes, exercise does burn calories, but considering how many calories we can easily consume, exercise doesn't burn enough of them to counterbalance our plentiful food supply. It is crucial for us to learn to value ourselves enough to not throw away valiant efforts to exercise by making frequent unwise eating choices.

One exciting benefit of exercise is that the more you exercise, the more fit you become, the more lean muscle tissue you develop, and therefore the more calories you burn during a workout. In addition, as you become better conditioned, your muscles adapt to using an enzyme that oxidizes fat—meaning you burn more fat during your workouts than an ordinary sedentary person.[13]

My point with all of this is that you have to balance the calories you eat with the calories you expend. If you were to eat only 1,000 calories per day of a fattening, unhealthy food like butter (don't try this at home) and your body expended 1,800 calories per day, then yes, you would lose weight, because you would not be consuming more than you expend. On the other hand, if you ate 3,000 calories per day of broccoli (you probably shouldn't try this at home either) and your body expended 1,800 calories per day, would you gain weight? The answer is absolutely yes. Granted, managing weight is not always that black-and-white because of hormonal, metabolic, and genetic factors. But the general rule still stands: *calories count.* That explains why many fad diets out there actually work—for a time. Promoters of fad diets won't admit it, but the reality is that most fad diets are just a tricky way to cut calories. Think about it: Is it easier to cut out a complete group of foods—like carbohydrates—or to spend the day counting the calories from each serving of food you eat? It is important for all of us to acknowledge that we can lose weight through fad diets—*unhealthfully.* Don't mortgage your health for a quick-fix weight-loss diet. We can manage our weight *healthfully*—by eating healthful foods in moderation (first, we need to learn some serious portion control) and by exercising regularly. Our bodies need all of the vitamins, minerals, phytochemicals, proteins, fats, and carbohydrates that are found in a variety of foods. Our bodies also need regular physical activity. Learning to balance all these things is the only way to live healthy and manage your weight for a lifetime.

Nobody is exempt from needing regular physical activity. And deep down, each of us has the ability and the emotional drive to exercise in some capacity. The benefits are priceless—if we can just make our precious physical, emotional, and spiritual health worthy of a mere thirty minutes per day.

## Notes

1. Jonathan Shaw, "The Deadliest Sin," *Harvard Magazine,* March–April 2004.

2. Jonathan Shaw, "The Deadliest Sin," *Harvard Magazine,* March–April 2004.

3. G. J. Balady, "Survival of the Fittest—More Evidence," *New England Journal of Medicine,* 2002; 346(11):852.

4. *Journal of Discourses,* 26 vols. (London: Latter-day Saints' Book Depot, 1854–86), 4:295.

5. Centers for Disease Control, www.wonder.cdc.gov/scripts/broker.exe.

6. *Dietary Guidelines for Americans 2005* (U.S. Department of Health and Human Services and the U.S. Department of Agriculture), chapter 4.

7. Bonnie Liebman, *Nutrition Action,* vol. 27 no. 1, January/February 2000 (Center for Science in the Public Interest).

8. *Dietary Guidelines for Americans 2005* (U.S. Department of Health and Human Services and the U.S. Department of Agriculture), chapter 4.

9. http://www.cdc.gov/nccdphp/dnpa/physical/measuring/perceived_exertion.htm.

10. Miriam Nelson, as quoted in *Nutrition Action Newsletter,* September 2004.

11. Bonnie Liebman, *Nutrition Action,* vol. 27 no. 1, January/February 2000 (Center for Science in the Public Interest), 4.

12. Bonnie Liebman, *Nutrition Action,* vol. 27 no. 1, January/February 2000 (Center for Science in the Public Interest), 4.

13. Bonnie Liebman, *Nutrition Action,* vol. 27 no. 1, January/February 2000 (Center for Science in the Public Interest), 4.

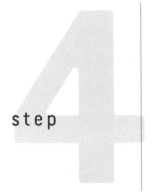

# Drink Good Cold Water

**KEY POINTS:**
Understanding Your Body's Water Needs | What Counts
As Water? | Water Needs During Exercise | Water Safety:
Tap or Bottled?

President Brigham Young said, "It is difficult to find anything more healthy to drink than good cold water, such as flows down to us from the springs and snows of our mountains. This is the beverage we should drink. It should be our drink at all times."[1]

Water is a vital nutrient for our bodies. Every cell, every tissue, every organ in our body needs water to function. Even your bones are made up of about 22 percent water. Water is vital to (1) regulate body temperature, (2) transport nutrients, (3) act as a medium for metabolic reactions, (4) carry waste away, and (5) provide form and structure to cells. Our bodies are largely made up of water, which accounts for approximately 55 to 65 percent of total body weight. For a 175-pound person, that equals approximately 12 to 14 gallons of water! Muscle holds more water than fat tissue, so athletes may have a higher percentage of body water than an elderly person (with a lower muscle mass), who may have much less. Our bodies can survive for weeks without food but only 10 days (in a moderate climate) without water. Children can survive only 5 days without water.[2] Unlike certain other nutrients (like body fat), your body doesn't store water for any special occasion. The water in your body is always "busy," involved in some active function. Therefore, we have to replace the water our body naturally loses every 24 hours. Losing body water is much more serious than most people think. Even losing just .5 percent will induce feelings of thirst. At a loss of 3 percent, physical performance is impaired. And a loss of 10 percent (15 pounds for a 150-pound person) causes severe disorders, muscle spasms, and delirium.[3]

However, getting too much water can also can be detrimental. Just as you can become dehydrated from lack of sufficient water, you can also suffer "water intoxication" from ingesting too much. Water intoxication is characterized by abdominal cramps, dizziness, lethargy, nausea, vomiting, or even convulsions and coma.[4]

Water balance is affected by two factors: water intake and water loss. Water intake is the water we consume through beverages and food. About 10 percent of our water intake comes from metabolic reactions inside our body, as water is produced from the digestion and metabolism of carbohydrates, proteins, and fats. We lose water through digestion, perspiration, and our respiratory tract. In normal temperatures, we can lose up to 10 cups of water per day. During hot weather or prolonged exercise, significantly higher amounts of water can be lost.

## How Much Water Does My Body Need?

In 2004, the Food and Nutrition Board of the Institute of Medicine, The National Academies released new guidelines for water intake which state that women should aim for approximately 90 ounces per day and men should aim for approximately 125 ounces per day. To some, that may sound like oodles of water, but in reality it is perfectly doable. First, solid foods also supply water so you can immediately cross off 16–24 ounces (or 2–3 cups) per day from solid foods. Second, the average portion size for water has even fallen into the "supersize" trap (which of course, is not all that bad)! If you actually drink from a now-miniature 8-ounce glass of water, that means you should drink 11–15 cups of water per day. Now for the rest of us, who usually drink from 12, 16, 20, or even 24-ounce glass or bottle of water, that means you should drink 4–6 *servings* of water per day. Oh, and let's not forget about the 32, 44, and 64-ounce refillable mugs that some of us tote around. Using these giant mugs can help you meet your water goals in one to three servings. Considering that almost none of the glasses or cups we drink from are only 8 ounces, it shouldn't be too hard to drink 90–125 ounces of water each day. Take a moment to check the label or volume capacity of your usual water container, then set a game plan for how many servings you need per day.

Thirst is generally but not always a reliable indicator of when you need to take a drink. In the case of infants, the elderly, those who are sick, and even hard-training athletes, thirst may not be a reliable indicator because their thirst sensation may be weakened. Conversely, thirst can even feel like hunger. So sometimes when we think we need to buy a Snickers bar or a bag of chips for the midafternoon munchies, our body is really just thirsty. A good rule of thumb is to drink a glass of water before giving in to a snack attack. Take a drink and see if the feeling goes away. If it doesn't, go for an apple or an alternative healthful snack.

If you are concerned about drinking enough water, simply check the color of your urine. Dark-colored urine means you need more water. (Keep in mind that vitamin supplements can darken urine.) Light or almost clear urine means you are getting an adequate amount.

## What Counts As Water?

Although water comes from many sources, the advice from Brigham Young hits the nail on the head: drink good, cold water. Plain water—it supplies no calories, no fat, and no cholesterol, and it comes right out of the tap. How much easier can it get? Your body needs water, pure and simple. Realistically, any fluid—milk, juice, or other beverages—count toward your daily water intake. Caffeinated beverages *do not* count; caffeine acts as a diuretic and stimulates the kidneys to excrete water instead of retain the water for body functions. Caffeine is found in many products: chocolate, beverages, and prescription or over-the-counter medications. The chart on this page shows the caffeine content of some common foods:

Solid foods are also a source of water for us. In fact, about 20 percent of the water we consume comes from solid foods. Foods such as celery, cabbage, lettuce, and watermelon are more than 90 percent water. Baked potatoes, cooked cereal, and milk are 75 percent to 90 percent water. Even meat, such as beef or chicken, is 60 to 65 percent water.[5] Oils are the exception at 0 percent water.

| FOOD | CAFFEINE (MG) |
|---|---|
| Chocolate bar (1.55 ounce) | 9 |
| Diet soda (12-oz. can) (32 fluid ounces) | 53 130 |
| Regular soda (12-oz. can) (32 fluid ounces) | 37–96 96–256 |
| Baking chocolate (2 squares) | 46 |
| Chocolate syrup (2 Tbsp.) | 5 |
| Hot cocoa mix (3 tsp.) | 5 |

*Source: USDA Agricultural Research Service Nutrient Database for Standard Reference, Release 17.*

# Water Needs During Exercise

Whether you are a conditioned athlete or a novice exerciser, you need to get enough fluids before, during, and after your workouts. Thirst is not always a reliable indicator of when you need to take a drink. Physical activity produces heat, which is then evaporated through the skin as sweat. Water lost through sweat needs to be replaced for the body to perform optimally during and after exercise. There are three simple rules to follow when exercising:

1. *Before:* Drink eight ounces of water fifteen to thirty minutes before you start.

2. *During:* Drink four to eight ounces of water every fifteen minutes during activity.

3. *After:* Drink a cup of water for every 250 calories you burn. If you sweat a lot, drink two to three cups of water for each pound lost during activity. You don't have to weigh yourself before and after every workout—maybe just try this once to see what kind of "sweater" you really are. If you lose one pound, then drink two to three cups to replace that loss. If you prefer not to weigh yourself, try to drink based on the estimated number of calories you burned. Or just play it safe and drink 8 to 16 ounces after a workout.

Water is the beverage of choice for any exercise session lasting less than one hour. If exercise is intense and lasts more than an hour, you may want to consider using a sports drink to help you keep up your energy level. Sports drinks also supply electrolytes—mainly sodium, chloride, and potassium—and help the body absorb more water. Your body does lose electrolytes during moderate exercise lasting less than one hour, but only in small amounts that are easily replaced by regular food. For rigorous, longer-lasting exercise sessions, sports drinks are a good choice because they replace electrolytes and have a lower sugar concentration that helps reduce the risk of stomach cramps or diarrhea that may occur when consuming a highly concentrated source of sugar (like fruit juice).

## Water Safety: Tap or Bottled?

Water comes in many forms. Tap water, bottled water, mineral water, purified water, sparkling water, and spring water are all forms of water available for us to drink. Is one form better than another? Not necessarily. Tap water is regulated by the Environmental Protection Agency (EPA), and bottled water is regulated by the Food and Drug Administration (FDA). Both forms of water are essentially safe. Most of us take for granted that we have drinkable water right from the tap! Nonetheless, there are contaminants in most of the water we drink. But rest assured, there are standards set forth and regulated by the EPA for the 80 different contaminants that may occur in drinking water. If you would like to find out about the water in your area, simply call the EPA Safe Drinking Hotline: 1-800-426-4791. If you want to take extra precautions with your tap water, you can try a home filter. But don't go broke thinking you always have to buy bottled water, because bottled and tap water are both regulated by the government. I personally like to be aware of but not become obsessive about such matters—there are contaminants everywhere, in food and water, in the air, and even on contact surfaces. I think we need to focus on the things we can control to improve our health and *not* on the things we can't control, such as environmental factors. Our bodies need water to survive, and that should be our first and primary concern.

At the grocery store, or in other food areas, you will see many different label names for bottled water. The Food and Drug Administration has established a "Standard of Identity" to define specific bottled-water products. Here's the rundown on what the different names mean:

*Spring water:* Flows to the earth naturally from formations beneath the ground. Most bottled water is spring water.

*Purified water:* Has gone through distillation, deionization, reverse osmosis, or other processes while also meeting the definition of purified water in the *United States Pharmacopoeia.*

*Mineral water:* Naturally contains dissolved minerals (like calcium and magnesium) at a standard level of 250 parts per million. Minerals may not be added by the manufacturer.

*Sparkling water:* Water that contains carbon dioxide gas; the carbon dioxide may be there originally or may be added back in after treatment, but the carbon dioxide must be at the same level as when the water emerged from the source. Seltzer and club soda are *not* considered sparkling water; they are soft drinks.

*Artesian water:* A specific type of water that comes from a well. The well must tap an aquifer, which is a water-bearing underground layer of rock or sand. The water level must stand at some point above the top of the aquifer.[6]

So there you have it. Current scinece, government agencies, and prophets of old all agree: water is an important nutrient for everyone. Deciphering label lingo, having too much information at your fingertips via the internet, and door-to-door salesmen can make somthing as simple as drinkig water seem overly complicated. The bottom line is to drink water instead of calorie-laden sugary soft drinks, juices, and fruit drinks. Drinking water should be one of the easiest steps in the Losing It program. In fact, go and get a drink of good cold water right now.

## Notes

1. *Journal of Discourses,* 26 vols. (London: Latter-day Saints' Book Depot, 1854–86), 12:122.
2. Kathleen L. Mahon and Sylvia Escott-Stump, *Krause's Food, Nutrition, and Diet Therapy,* 9th ed. (Philadelphia: W.B. Saunders, 1996), 168, 169.
3. Kathleen L. Mahon and Sylvia Escott-Stump, *Krause's Food, Nutrition, and Diet Therapy,* 9th ed. (Philadelphia: W.B. Saunders, 1996), 168, 169.
4. *Taber's Cyclopedic Medical Dictionary,* 17th ed. (Philadephia: F.A. Davis Company, 1993).
5. Kathleen L. Mahon and Sylvia Escott-Stump, *Krause's Food, Nutrition, and Diet Therapy,* 9th ed. (Philadelphia: W. B. Saunders, 1996), 171.
6. International Bottle Water Association. http://www.bottledwater.org/public/BWFactsHome_Main.htm

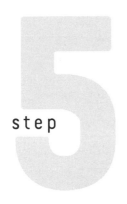

# Give It Time and Believe in Yourself

**KEY POINTS:**

Setting Realistic Goals | Understanding Why We Typically Fail | Overcoming Barriers to Exercise | Overcoming Barriers to Healthy Eating | Finding That Missing Spark: Motivation! | Last but Not Least: Believe in Yourself

This chapter is the hardest. It's hard to be patient. It's hard to be positive about yourself. And it's really hard to change. Think about it: If it were easy to change, you would have done so already. If you want to change something about yourself, what do you do? Set a goal! Health-oriented goals take time. If you want results that last beyond six months, you have to accept that maintainable, lifelong changes don't happen overnight. If you want to be healthy, then you need to work each and every day—not just for 6, 8, or 12 weeks. Be patient and take one day at a time.

## Setting Realistic Goals

There are five crucial steps to achieving and maintaining health-oriented goals:

1. Gain knowledge. Your mind and spirit have to clearly understand the risks of not changing and the benefits of making a change. Your mind has to understand why change is necessary.

2. Clearly define a realistic goal. It could be to buy 100 percent whole-wheat bread

instead of white, or it could be to lose 25 pounds in 12 weeks (which is a sensible 2-pound loss per week).

3. Be patient. Positive change takes time. Too many times, I have seen people give up when results were just around the corner. Not all health benefits are visible in the mirror. Over a six-week period, you may not have lost all the inches you wanted to lose, but, for example, your blood pressure may have improved—which is a very rewarding benefit. High blood pressure carries no symptoms but can yield devastating results. When you really think about it, what's more important: healthy, functioning, life-giving organs, like your heart and lungs, or an exterior appearance?

4. Expect to lapse, relapse, and even collapse. Occasionally, you may "lapse" by splurging on an unhealthy meal or missing a workout. Sometimes this can turn into a "relapse" and go on for an entire day, several days, or even weeks. Sometimes you may experience a full-blown "collapse"—meaning your mind tells you to completely give up on exercise and eating right. Regardless of when, where, or how often these feelings come up, there are two words that will always get you out of the going-nowhere rut: *Start again.* Don't ever throw your health-related goals and aspirations by the wayside just because of a few rough days. Just start again. Lapse, relapse, and, yes, even collapse are normal and perhaps even necessary parts of making permanent, lifelong changes. Always remember what Mary Pickford said: You may have a fresh start at any moment you choose, for this thing we call failure is not the falling down, but the staying down."

5. Ready! Set! Commit! I admit, making *lifelong* changes can sound a little overwhelming. So the basis of the "Losing It" program (outlined in the last section of this book) is to start by committing to follow the program six days per week for eight weeks. The "Five Keys to Successful Weight Loss That Work"—which

are simple yet essential in achieving health-oriented goals—are incorporated into the eight-week program. Commitment to your personal health is crucial. And I am not talking about adding another project to your to-do list and becoming an all-star multitasker. Just going through the motions, without really committing yourself, is a waste of time. We often give our best effort to keep our word when dealing with others—so why not for ourselves? Be true to yourself and keep your word to yourself. Always think about your real purpose in life and why you want to become a healthier person. "Into your hands will be placed the exact results of your own thoughts."[1]

## Understanding Why We Typically Fail

I think sometimes our attempts to change our health habits fail because we don't take our own personal health seriously enough. Many of us, although not in the best of health, are getting by just fine. So it is easy to give up and say, "Oh, forget it. I tried and failed." The problem with our society is that the consequences of poor health are sometimes camouflaged by aging, random disease, genetics, or other uncontrollable factors. High blood pressure, high cholesterol, weak bones, lack of energy, or even lack of strength to play with a child are all good examples of how poor health can be a "silent offender"; you may feel just fine, but do you really understand how much better and stronger you could be? Do you know that simple lifestyle choices could add years to your life, giving you more time to accomplish the things you were sent here to do? Now of course, living healthy doesn't guarantee a life free of disease, pain, or early death. However, we certainly have enough research to back up the fact that *not* living healthy does raise your risk for disease, pain, and early death.

Also contributing to our supposed failure to attempt or stick to a health-improvement program are common excuses or myths such as the following:

- "Weight gain is inevitable with age."

- "I'm too old to start an exercise program."

- "I'm too out of shape to start an exercise program."

- "If I can't exercise regularly, why even start?"

- "I can't be fit if I'm overweight."

None of these statements is valid or true. Even though we do naturally lose muscle as we age, and therefore gain some weight as the result of a lower metabolic rate, that certainly doesn't mean weight gain is inevitable. It just means you have to fight for your health. And the truth is, we all have to fight for our health—children, teens, adults, and seniors. Each stage in life has its own trials. And at each stage in life, our health is important.

Taking things to the extreme is another reason we why seem to fail. If your goals are too restrictive (like eliminating healthful food groups completely) or too unrealistic (like living on diet shakes or special diet foods), the result is often a breakdown. You can only manipulate yourself for so long. Likewise, continual unhealthful eating patterns and sedentary behavior also have negative consequences. These are essentially addictive behaviors. The word "addictive" sounds harsh, but it is true. Good things can be addictive, sometimes in a good or bad way. Fatty food tastes good. Reclining on the couch without lifting a finger can feel like heaven. And although these things certainly aren't bad once in a while, they can be detrimental to your health when taken to the extreme. Any behavior or habit taken to the extreme is unhealthy for you—mind, body, and spirit.

In order to avoid the "failure" trap, remember these three points:

1. Take your health seriously. That doesn't mean you can't enjoy a little flexibility with your habits or indulge a little here and there. Taking your health seriously means that you have the determination to get back on your program as soon

as possible. If you have a crazy day, then start again the next day—don't just give up.

2. Don't fall victim to the common myths of health-related change. Too old, too overweight, too out of shape, not enough time—none of these is a good excuse for not even trying to make small changes.

3. Avoid extremism. Use moderation, sensibility, balance, and flexibility. That is what life is all about; why should your diet and exercise habits be any different?

# Overcoming Barriers to Exercise

Since the statistics clearly show that the majority of us are overweight, too inactive, and too skimpy on healthful food choices, I have concluded that we all share a similar burden: barriers. Let's start with barriers to exercise. Realistically, we can get adequate exercise at any time and any place. The key is to find something you enjoy—because if you don't enjoy it, you won't stick with it. There are pros and cons to every exercise environment; however, the next few pages provide tips for success in any environment.

## Working Out at Home

Don't feel obligated to go to a gym; working out at home is a great place to start—and finish! Your home is convenient, private, flexible, affordable, and time saving. You don't have to sit in traffic or make an appointment, and you don't have to find a babysitter. In fact, working out at home will teach your kids healthy habits too.

Here are the basic tips for a successful home workout program:

- *Reveille, Reveille, Reveille.* I can't emphasis this enough. Let's face it: If you plan your workout for later in the day, it won't happen. Too many distractions will pop up, and pretty soon you'll be sitting in front of the TV with a quart of ice cream, thinking, "Oh well, I missed my workout today, but I will work out tomorrow." (I know, because I have done this myself.) But seriously, if you think you're not a morning person because you can't get to bed early, just go to bed late and get up early for about a week. At that point, going to bed thirty minutes earlier will be much easier.

- *Invest in some good equipment.* Of course, you can work out at home without spending a dime. But for optimal results, it is best to have access to some home exercise equipment. Here are a few of the options:

  - *Stability ball and a resistance tube or hand weights (www.workoutwarehouse.com or www.proform.com.).* A stability ball is a great way to get a fun yet effective strength-training workout. You can tone and strengthen your body and boost your metabolism with these two simple pieces of equipment. (See the appendix for specific exercises.)

  - *Treadmill (www.nordictrack.com or www.proform.com).* Americans spend significantly more on treadmills than any other piece of fitness equipment—and for good reason. Treadmills continually emerge as the winner for burning the most calories in the least amount of time.[2] Treadmills have a motor that essentially drives you to challenge your body to work at an appropriate level. With other pieces of equipment, it is easy to just ho-hum along at a pace that is comfortable—sometimes too comfortable. Additionally, with a treadmill you can walk at .1 mile per hour or run at a heart-pounding 12 miles per hour—which accommodates everyone from the beginner to the elite athlete. Most treadmills now have power incline, which increases the intensity of the workout without having to run or jog—a great benefit for delicate knees, hips, and backs.

  - *Bike or elliptical (www.nordictrack.com or www.proform.com).* Bikes and ellipticals have come a long way in the past ten years, and both provide a great workout with little impact to knees and joints. For bikes, you can choose from an upright bike (similar to a real bike) or a recumbent bike (similar to sitting in a chair). Most models have a resistance feature, which means anyone, from the rehab patient to the elite athlete, can get a challenging, efficient workout.

- *Strength machine. (www.workoutwarehouse.com or www.thecoremaster.com)* If you have extra space, a strength machine is a great investment. For those who are new to strength training, a machine can be safer and make it easier to learn the exercises. However, most people get along fine with a few dumbbells, a stability ball, or a bench. Many of us are enticed by super-cheap, perfect-for-the-problem-area "abdominal" machines. However, you can always do good old abdominal crunches on a stability ball or the floor, and several other exercises are just as effective. (See specific examples in the appendix.) Machines or exercise programs that work the "core" muscles instead of just "abs" are a much better investment. Your core consists of approximately 35 muscles that attach to your spine and pelvis. These muscles are essentially your powerhouse, the centerpiece for almost every move you make. Overall, eating healthy, getting regular aerobic activity, and strengthening the core muscles is the best way to lose excess abdominal fat.

## Finding Time to Exercise

Exercising won't just happen; you'll have to make time for it. Here are a few tips you may find helpful:

- *Plan ahead to avoid distractions.* Try not to schedule your home workout during the busiest part of the day. If you have kids, make sure they have a project to work on or something to do before you start. Maybe turn the ringer off on your phone. You can return calls in 30 minutes. Let others in the house know that this is a priority for you.

- *Use motivating music, read a book, or watch TV.* Music with a steady, uplifting beat can do wonders for a workout. Reading a good book can make the time fly. Find anything that keeps you motivated and use it!

- *Look for opportunities to do two things at once.* Is there a TV program you watch every day? The morning or evening news? If there are any activities that regularly take up part of your day, try to combine them and your workout time into one task. For example, there are days when I may have missed the chance to work out in the morning. After working at the office all day, the last thing I want to do is leave my kids so I can go work out. So sometimes I take them to the park, and you know what I do? I run laps around the playground while my kids play. If that idea seems too quirky, try taking a soccer ball or Frisbee to the park. Maybe play tag with your children or grandchildren. Don't ever let feelings of insecurity (if your soccer skills are as pitiful as mine) stop you from seizing a perfect opportunity to get off the park bench and get moving.

- *Go for variety.* Your body adapts to doing the same thing every day, so don't be afraid to shake up your workouts. Try walking, jogging, biking, strength training, or even vigorous housecleaning to keep things exciting.

## Working Out at a Gym

- *Use your membership.* Too many people sign up for a health club membership, pay for it, and then never use it. Surprisingly enough, some of these people even wonder *why* they never got any results.

- *Don't be afraid to try new things.* Many health clubs offer great variety—weights, aerobics, racquetball, tennis, basketball, and swimming. Don't let yourself feel insecure. Everyone there is trying to do the same thing you are—become healthier. If you have questions about how to use a specific piece of equipment, ask a personal trainer. Even if you have to pay for one session, it is for your health—and I think that is always a good investment.

- *Don't let a little muscle soreness scare you off.* I have worked in a health club since the age of 18. I can't tell you how many times I have seen new people come into the club, work way too hard, get sore muscles, and never come back. So first, try not to kill yourself the first few times you go to the club. Second, remember that muscle soreness is okay. You shouldn't have to deal with sore muscles after every workout. But as your body adapts to new things, a little soreness will come and go.

## Working Out While Traveling

Just because you're away from home doesn't mean it's okay to skip working out. Here are some ideas that will help you stay healthy, even while traveling:

- *Take a resistance tube with you.* With the exercises outlined in the back of this book, you can use a resistance tube to get a good workout in the privacy and convenience of your hotel room.

- *Ask the hotel if they have a fitness center.* Many hotels have a complimentary small fitness room with a few treadmills, bikes, and sometimes hand weights or strength machines. If a hotel offers this service, use it! If the hotel charges for the fitness center and you are required to travel for your employer, ask your employer about paying the hotel fitness center fee. With the rising burden of health-care costs in America, I think many corporations will give your request serious consideration.

- *Exaggerate everyday activities.* If you don't have the time to get a structured workout during your travels, then get all you can out of your typical everyday activities. For example, take the stairs at every opportunity, park as far away as possible, take a five-minute walk here and there, or even use restrooms at the other end of the building.

- *Make sensible eating choices.* If your busy time on the road doesn't accommodate physical activity, then don't let eating too many calories compound the problem. Because you are not expending enough calories, you should make extra efforts to eat less.

## Working Out When Money Is Tight

Even if you're counting pennies, there are still ways to exercise, and many of them are free!

- *Ask for healthful birthday or holiday gifts.* Exercise equipment, hand weights, new exercise shoes, or even a trial health club membership don't have to be expensive.
- *Sign up for community sports.* You never know, you might become the next star of the team. If not, you still might find a new activity that you enjoy!
- *Try a simple home workout video.* Home exercise videos can cost as little as $10.00. For such a small expense, this is a very worthwhile investment.
- *Exaggerate everyday activities.* Be more active around the house. Vacuum vigorously, mop the floors, or refinish a piece of furniture. Lose your TV remote. Wash your dishes by hand. Do simple exercises like push-ups, squats, or stomach crunches. You can even walk up and down your stairs for a workout.
- Walk, jog, or run outside for 30 minutes on most days of the week.

## Overcoming a Lack of Energy

Just don't have the "oomph" to get started? Think "mind over matter." The sad truth is that the less physical activity you get, the more energy you lack. Exercise is rejuvenating. Often, just changing your clothes and tying your shoelaces is the hardest part. Once you get going and your heart starts pumping, you will feel a new energy flowing through your body. You just have to find a way to make yourself take the first step—like getting off the couch. If you can't find the energy to start a structured workout, then take small steps to become more active throughout the day. Bit by bit, these short bouts of activity will help you begin to boost your energy level. For example:

- *Bicycle or walk to do errands or visit friends.*
- *Make family time more active.* Go bowling or dancing, play team sports, or take a walk instead of going to the movies.
- *Exaggerate everyday activities.* Be more active around the house. Vacuum vigorously, mop the floors, or refinish a piece of furniture. Lose your TV remote. Wash your dishes by hand.
- *Recruit a friend to work out with you.* No doubt about it, a workout buddy helps you stick with it. Knowing that you have an appointment to exercise and that someone else is counting on you to show up can make all the difference in the world.
- *Keep your gym shoes or gym bag visible.* This is a simple but subtle reminder that can help you find the energy to get moving.

## Overcoming Barriers to Healthy Eating

Recent research from the United States Department of Agriculture (1999 to 2000) found that 74 percent of Americans had a diet that "needs improvement." Sixteen percent of us had a "poor diet," and a mere 10 percent of us had a "good diet."[3] Obviously, eating healthy has gotten harder in this fast-paced society. Here are a few more tips (in addition to the many tips listed in chapter 2) that can help you stay on track with your healthy-eating goals:

- Grab a few pieces of fresh fruit (apples, oranges, pears, etc.) on your way out the door. Keep them in the car to tide you over when hunger strikes on the road. This tactic is great for hungry kids too.

- Eat a light breakfast or exercise an extra 15 to 30 minutes if you know you are going to eat a heavy lunch or dinner for a special occasion.

- Eat snacks like pretzels from a plate, or place a single serving in a sandwich baggie instead of eating straight from the big bag. This will help you consume only one portion instead of mindless handful after handful from the bag.

- If you have to eat out often, try to eat only half the served portion—or share with a friend.

- Think small. Keep portions under control at home and on the road.

- Split a must-have dessert with a friend (or two friends).

- Read food labels.

- Use spinach on sandwiches and in salads instead of pale iceberg lettuce.

- Put all snack foods, junk foods, or tempting foods in your cupboard and out of sight. Put fruits, vegetables, and healthful snacks on the counter or in a visible spot in the refrigerator.

- Use high-fiber (three to five grams per serving) dry cereal as a snack instead of potato chips. Pour a one-cup serving into a baggie or bowl, and then put the large box of cereal out of sight.

- Keep single-serving containers of yogurt on hand for a calcium-rich snack.

- Pack away a few pieces of fresh fruit or single-serving cereal boxes into your suitcase when you are going on the road.

- Keep fat-free single-serving bags of popcorn handy at work or home for a quick snack.

- If you find yourself craving a fattening or salty snack, have a tall glass of water and go find something productive to do: vacuum, call a friend, or go for a walk. Just find something to get your mind off food.

- Cut out sugar! 1 teaspoon of sugar for every 4 grams of sugar listed on a food label. A 20-ounce soda has at least *17 teaspoons* of sugar!

# Finding That Missing Spark: Motivation!

Taking the time to gain more knowledge about fitness and nutrition is an essential first step in achieving good health. But that is only the beginning. You must also find the motivation within yourself to put that knowledge into practice. Through my experience in this industry, I have found that lack of motivation is the number-one reason people quit exercising or give up new eating habits. The reason: motivation is like dust in the wind; it changes from one moment to the next.

Many times, after spending a full hour with clients, I finally see it in the clients' eyes: They are motivated. They feel powerful and in control of their eating and exercise habits. They are ready to take on the world. Then they get into their cars and start to drive home, and guess what they run into? Bright lights proclaiming "Grab a delicious double-patty melt" or "Hungry? Try a triple-chocolate, peanut butter, fudge-ripple, cookie-covered ice-cream cone" or possibly "Don't cook. Pick up a thick-crust double-cheese and meat pizza."

Okay, so maybe this is a slight exaggeration, but temptations like this are certainly all around us. It is absolutely necessary for you to find something—an emotional hook—that will give you the strength to overcome temptation. This is important because the surplus of mouth-watering food and the ease of our leisure is not going to change. In fact, I don't know if we will ever live in a world where we don't have to make a conscious effort to fight for our health. Motivation is driven by a want or need that will cause you to act. You need to ask yourself what it is that you really want, and you need to keep that specific goal in mind over the next few weeks or months. That is your motivation.

When thinking about your personal goals and your purpose for wanting to become a healthier person, it is important to set a realistic goal, which we've talked about. Now you have to fine-tune your goal. By this I mean you have to clearly define it: "I want to lose 12 pounds in 12 weeks." You also need to clearly define what benefit or reward you will receive: "I will have the energy to go on a bike ride with my kids." We all need something to strive for, and it helps to get specific. Here are a few of the rewards that may come from engaging in a healthy eating and exercise program (and no, looking like Barbie is not an option):

- Feel better.
- Lose weight, if necessary.
- Become stronger for physical activities.
- Become stronger to carry a bag of groceries, pick up a child, or perform activities of daily living.
- Enjoy time with family and friends.
- Be physically and emotionally strong to raise a family, protect growing children, and care for loved ones.
- Sleep better.
- Feel emotionally stable (reduce anxiety, stress, depression, and mood swings).
- Reduce the severity of a disease (arthritis, heart disease, diabetes, high blood pressure) and possibly reduce the need for medications.
- Live longer.
- Improve self-confidence and self-reliance.
- Be an example to children or loved ones.
- Be healthy in order to fulfill your eternal purpose in life.

Setting a goal toward one of these rewards instead of gaining a specific look will help you to be successful. I don't recommend setting goals around a look (sorry, Barbie), because attaining a certain body type, look, or size is not always realistic. Regardless of how you look, employing habits of regular exercise and healthy eating are good for you, and it's a shame that people sometimes throw healthy habits out the window just because they didn't turn into a 5'10" 110-pound genetic abnormality seen only on magazine covers.

## Keeping a Journal

Keeping a journal can be one of the most eye-opening, mind-boggling things you'll ever experience. It is also one of the greatest motivational tools ever. Sometimes when we think we've been "so good," we really haven't. It's easy to forget the cookie we grabbed earlier, the handful of candy, or the workout we thought we missed only the past two days but really the entire last week.

Keeping a journal helps you to boldly see what you *really* do—instead of what you *think* you do. I'm one of those people who does an extremely poor job of balancing my checkbook. And every month when I get my statement, I think, "There is no way I spent that much money." I then comb through the bank statement with absolute certainty that somewhere on that page is an error made by the bank. Of course, I am wrong; we all know that the bank doesn't make mistakes. The same can be true of our eating and exercise habits. Sometimes, we just have to see our actions on paper in order to realize that we need to try harder. Likewise, sometimes seeing our success on paper can be as motivational and rewarding as anything else.

On the following page is a sample journal page that you may wish to copy and use over the next several weeks.

# Last but Not Least: Believe in Yourself

Have you ever had someone say, "You're not strong enough," "You're not smart enough," or, "It's hopeless—you're just too out of shape"? Who was it that said those terrible things? If you're like most people, it was *you*—you were the person who uttered those harsh words to yourself! Often, I think we say things to ourselves that we wouldn't say to our worst enemy. We can impose limits on ourselves better than anybody else can.

| Health and Fitness Goal: 30 minutes of aerobic or strength training 5 days per week. 1,900-calorie diet 5 days per week. | | | |
|---|---|---|---|
| **FITNESS** | **MEALS** | **SNACKS** | **NOTES** |
| **MONDAY** ☐ I met my fitness goal today. Aerobic Strength | ☐ I met my meal goal today. ☐ Breakfast (400 calories) ☐ Lunch (400 calories) ☐ Dinner (500 calories) | ☐ I met my snack goal today. Snacks (goal:_____) | |
| **TUESDAY** ☐ I met my fitness goal today. Aerobic Strength | ☐ I met my meal goal today. ☐ Breakfast (400 calories) ☐ Lunch (400 calories) ☐ Dinner (500 calories) | ☐ I met my snack goal today. Snacks (goal:_____) | |
| **WEDNESDAY** ☐ I met my fitness goal today. Aerobic Strength | ☐ I met my meal goal today. ☐ Breakfast (400 calories) ☐ Lunch (400 calories) ☐ Dinner (500 calories) | ☐ I met my snack goal today. Snacks (goal:_____) | |
| **THURSDAY** ☐ I met my fitness goal today. Aerobic Strength | ☐ I met my meal goal today. ☐ Breakfast (400 calories) ☐ Lunch (400 calories) ☐ Dinner (500 calories) | ☐ I met my snack goal today. Snacks (goal:_____) | |
| **FRIDAY** ☐ I met my fitness goal today. Aerobic Strength | ☐ I met my meal goal today. ☐ Breakfast (400 calories) ☐ Lunch (400 calories) ☐ Dinner (500 calories) | ☐ I met my snack goal today. Snacks (goal:_____) | |
| **SATURDAY** ☐ I met my fitness goal today. Aerobic Strength | ☐ I met my meal goal today. ☐ Breakfast (400 calories) ☐ Lunch (400 calories) ☐ Dinner (500 calories) | ☐ I met my snack goal today. Snacks (goal:_____) | |
| **SUNDAY** ☐ I met my fitness goal today. Aerobic Strength | ☐ I met my meal goal today. ☐ Breakfast (400 calories) ☐ Lunch (400 calories) ☐ Dinner (500 calories) | ☐ I met my snack goal today. Snacks (goal:_____) | |

Now, on the flip side, think about something you've done in the past that you are proud of. It took a lot of determination, a lot of discipline, and a lot of hard work. Who was it that gave you the strength to accomplish that great task? Ahhh. You again! Do you fully realize your potential? Look deep inside yourself. You have the power, that constant driving spirit, to accomplish anything you want. There is not a single soul with more power than you to persuade yourself. You will never realize that power unless you at least give it a try! Sometimes, we may need to ask the Lord to help us find the strength to accomplish a difficult task, which is perfectly normal. I believe the Lord can help us find the strength within ourselves to do what we were created to do.

Believing in something and putting good intentions into daily practice are completely dependent on each other. For example, do you value yourself enough to believe that you have the right to be kept safe? How do you act on that belief? By buckling your seatbelt? By avoiding a tumultuous walk across six lanes of freeway traffic? Do you see how easy it can be to "just do it" when you really believe in the cause? The bottom line is that you have to believe in yourself, respect yourself, and value yourself enough to make health a priority in your life. If you truly believe you deserve to be healthy and that good health is beneficial to you and your family, then you will act accordingly. If you do not believe in yourself, that too is changeable.

Even if you are not sure at this point, take the first step. Get on the right path. You might progress only one tiny inch at time. But at least you are on the right path—a path that can enhance every moment of your life. Maybe you even need to get down on your knees; just as the Spirit reveals the truthfulness of the gospel, I believe with all my heart that if you ask, the Spirit will also confirm the fact that the Lord loves you and wants you to be healthy—he wants you to have the strength to do great things.

Now *that* is something to believe in.

## Notes

1. James Allen, *As a Man Thinketh*.
2. A. I. Zeni, M. D. Hoffman, and P. S. Clifford, "Energy Expenditure with Indoor Exercise Machines," *Journal of the American Medical Association*, May 8, 1996, vol. 275, no. 18.
3. http://www.usda.gov/cnpp/Pubs/HEI/HEI99–00report.pdf

# The Losing It Program

**KEY POINTS:**

Action 1: The Flexible Meal Planner

Action 2: Cardiovascular Exercise

Action 3: Strength Training

Action 4: Commit

The Losing It program is essentially a daily planning guide that helps you put the "Five Keys to Successful Weight Loss That Work" into action. Before we get specific about designing a program that works for you, take a moment to fully understand what the Losing It program requires you to complete:

*Action 1:* Use the flexible meal planner six days per week to help you eat sensibly and healthfully.

*Action 2:* Complete at least 30 minutes of cardiovascular exercise on most days of the week.

*Action 3:* Complete at least 30 minutes of strength training two to three times per week.

*Action 4:* Commit to the program six days per week for at least eight weeks. (That's right, you get one day off! You can do anything for six days, right?)

## The Losing It Program: Action #1 The Flexible Meal Planner

The Flexible Meal Planner (starting on page 137) should be used 6 days per week to help you make healthy choices. The Flexible Meal Planner is essentially a list of calorie-controlled choices for breakfast, lunch, dinner, and snacks. The Flexible Meal Planner includes:

- 21 Breakfast options at 400 calories each
- 21 Lunch options at 400 calories each

- 21 Dinner options at 500 calories each
  - 8 Gourmet Options with healthy recipes included (see page181).
  - 9 Quick & Easy options that don't require a recipe because they are familiar foods and easy to prepare.
- 230+ Snack options from which to choose
- 30+ Healthy and delicious recipes that are easy to prepare

In order to use the Flexible Meal Planner, follow these simple steps:

1. First, forget about your past exercise habits and focus on the future. What are you going to do for the next eight to twelve weeks? Now, decide which level of activity fits your commitment to the Losing It program:

**Sedentary**: no physical activity other than the light activity associated with typical day-to-day life. (*Remember, exercise is a vital part of the program. This should only be an option for those with special medical concerns or other circumstances in which regular exercise may not be appropriate.*)

**Moderately active**: physical activity equivalent to walking 1.5 to 3 miles (or 15–45 minutes) at 3 to 4 miles per hour on most days of the week.

**Active**: physical activity equivalent to walking more than 3 miles (or 30 to 90 minutes) at 3 to 4 miles per hour on most days of the week.

(*Physical activity classifications are adapted from The Dietary Guidelines for Americans 2005 Table 3. "Estimated Calorie Requirements for Each Gender and Age Group at Three Levels of Physical Activity.")*

2. Second, use one of the charts below to find your daily calorie budget. Each chart is specific for gender, goal (weight loss or weight maintenance), age and activity level. This is the **maximum** number of calories you should strive to eat each day.

3. Third, put it all together. The calories from breakfast (400), lunch (400) and dinner (500) adds up to 1300 calories per day. That means you should subtract the number 1300 from your daily calorie budget to find out how many calories you can have in snacks per day.

For example, a 45-year old active female who wants to lose weight has a calorie budget of 1700 calories per day. Subtract 1300 and that means she can have up to 400 calories per day in snacks . . . spread throughout the day, or for certain high-calorie unmentionables, maybe all at once (only once and a while please!).

| WOMEN DAILY CALORIE BUDGET for a Weight Loss of 1 to 2 pounds per week | | | |
|---|---|---|---|
| Age | Sedentary | Moderately Active | Active |
| 19-30 | 1500 | 1700 | 1900 |
| 31-50 | 1400 | 1500 | 1700 |
| 51+ | 1400 | 1500 | 1500 – 1700 |

| MEN DAILY CALORIE BUDGET for a Weight Loss of 1 to 2 pounds per week | | | |
|---|---|---|---|
| Age | Sedentary | Moderately Active | Active |
| 18-30 | 1900 | 2100 – 2300 | 2500 |
| 31-50 | 1700 | 1900 – 2100 | 2300 – 2500 |
| 51+ | 1500 | 1700 – 1900 | 1900 – 2300 |

| WOMEN DAILY CALORIE BUDGET for Weight Maintenance[b] | | | |
|---|---|---|---|
| Age | Sedentary | Moderately Active | Active |
| 18-30 | 2000 | 2000 – 2200 | 2400 |
| 31-50 | 1800 | 2000 | 2200 |
| 51+ | 1600 | 1800 | 2000 – 2200 |

| MEN DAILY CALORIE BUDGET for Weight Maintenance[b] | | | |
|---|---|---|---|
| Age | Sedentary | Moderately Active | Active |
| 18-30 | 2400 | 2600 – 2800 | 3000 |
| 31-50 | 2200 | 2400 – 2600 | 2800 – 3000 |
| 51+ | 2000 | 2200 – 2400 | 2400 – 2800 |

(*b Dietary Guidelines for Americans 2005 Table 3. "Estimated Calorie Requirements for Each Gender and Age Group at Three Levels of Physical Activity" Levels based on Estimated Energy Requirements (EER) from the Institute of Medicine Dietary Reference Intakes macronutrients report, 2002, calculated by gender, age, and activity level for reference-sized individuals. "Reference size," as determined by IOM is based on median height and weight for that height to give a BMI of 21.5 for adult females and 22.5 for adult males.)*

## A Few Key Points Regarding Daily Calorie Budgets:

- I like to use the term "calorie budget" because a give-and-take attitude is absolutely necessary when it comes to controlling food intake. If you eat too much at one meal, you need to eat less at the next meal. If you have a high-calorie day, you need to balance it with a low-calorie day. If your calorie budget allows for 300 calories per day in snacks and you eat all 300 calories in two enormous bites of chocolate cake, then you don't get to eat any more snacks for the rest of the day! And if you lose complete control and have a crazy, incalculable day, then *be strong* and eat less the next day (I sometimes even skip breakfast . . . yet, try not skip meals more than once a week) or workout for an *extra* 15 to 30 minutes to make up for it.

- You may find that your recommended calorie budget is simply too high or too low. Remember that these are *average* recommendations for healthy individuals. Listen to your body. If you are starving, you may need to add an extra *healthy* snack or two. If you are stuffed, certainly don't eat more just because your meal plan says so. Even if I were to give you a more precise recommendation for your daily calorie needs (which requires more detailed evaluation), it is virtually impossible to stick to that exact number. To elaborate, think of this example: I can buy two apples from the same store. One may be larger and provide 160 calories, and one may be smaller and provide 80 calories. The bottom line is to keep portions small and remember that these numbers are "averages." The types of foods you choose to eat are important. Counting every single calorie that comes near your mouth is not.

- If your daily calorie budget seems to low, remember that it is okay to aim low. Most of us eat much more than we think. Ironically, most of us think we are much more active than we actually are.

## Final Meal-Planning Tips

Remember, this meal plan is designed to be flexible and to help you control calorie intake. "On the Go" options may not be as healthy and therefore should be used sparingly;

they are there simply because we lead busy lives, and pretending that we don't dine "on the go" won't help any of us get healthier. The snack options are also designed in this way—meaning that some options are more healthful than others. Try to choose fruits, vegetables, nuts, and whole grains as often as possible. Splurging on chocolate, ice cream, baked goods, or movie snacks is also a normal part of our lives. These items are listed as snack options but should be used sparingly. Pay attention to the calories per serving on these types of "indulgence" foods so you can learn how to counterbalance higher-calorie food choices with lighter meals or extra exercise. Here are a few additional tips to help you succeed with this meal plan and make it part of your lifelong path to good health:

1. Balance food and exercise, large portions with small portions, high-fat entrees with low-fat entrees.
2. Think small on portions.
3. Think big on vegetables.
4. Go for variety.
5. Be flexible.
6. Be sensible.
7. Be realistic.
8. Use moderation in all good things.

## Action 2: Cardiovascular Exercise

Remember to try to get in at least 30 to 60 minutes of cardiovascular exercise on most days of the week. If you currently exercise on most days of the week, then good for you! However, if you no longer feel challenged by your regular workouts, then set a goal to try something new—shake things up a bit. If you do not currently engage in regular cardiovascular activity, use the Aerobic Exercise: Calorie Expenditure Chart to pick something you will enjoy, and then go for it!

| AEROBIC EXERCISE: CALORIE EXPENDITURE CHART | | |
|---|---|---|
| Activity | Calories burned per minute | Calories burned in 30 minutes |
| Aerobic Dancing (high impact) | 10 | 300 |
| Aerobic Dancing (low impact) | 7 | 214 |
| Basketball (nongame) | 9 | 257 |
| Basketball (shooting baskets) | 6 | 193 |
| Bicycling (< 10 mph) leisure, or for pleasure | 6 | 171 |
| Bicycling (12–13.9 mph) leisure, moderate effort | 11 | 343 |
| Bicycling (14–15.9 mph) racing or leisure, fast vigorous effort | 14 | 428 |
| Bicycling (mountain) | 12 | 364 |
| Bicycling (stationary) | 7 | 214 |
| Bowling | 4 | 129 |
| Child care: (standing) bathing, grooming, feeding, dressing | 5 | 150 |
| Circuit Training | 11 | 343 |
| Cleaning, heavy (washing car, mopping, washing windows) | 6 | 193 |
| Cleaning, light (dusting, sweeping, straightening up, vacuuming) | 4 | 107 |
| Cooking or Food Preparation | 4 | 107 |
| Food Shopping, with grocery cart | 5 | 150 |
| Gardening (digging, spading, filling garden) | 7 | 214 |
| Gardening (planting seeds) | 6 | 171 |
| Gardening (weeding, cultivating garden) | 6 | 193 |
| Golf (carrying clubs) | 8 | 236 |
| Golf (using a power cart) | 5 | 150 |
| Hiking (cross country) | 9 | 257 |
| Ice Skating | 10 | 300 |
| Ironing | 3 | 99 |
| Lying Quietly (watching television) | 1 | 39 |
| Making bed | 3 | 86 |
| Mowing Lawn (walking, power mower) | 6 | 193 |
| Playing Piano or Organ | 4 | 107 |
| Running Cross Country | 13 | 386 |

| AEROBIC EXERCISE: CALORIE EXPENDITURE CHART | | |
|---|---|---|
| **Activity** | **Calories burned per minute** | **Calories burned in 30 minutes** |
| Running, 5 mph (12 min. mile) | 11 | 343 |
| Running, 6 mph (10 min. mile) | 14 | 428 |
| Running, 7.5 mph (8 min. mile) | 18 | 536 |
| Running, 10 mph (6 min. mile) | 23 | 685 |
| Scrubbing Floors (on hands and knees) | 8 | 236 |
| Sitting Quietly (reading, riding in a car, listening to a lecture or music) | 1 | 43 |
| Skiing, downhill (light effort) | 7 | 214 |
| Skiing, downhill (moderate effort) | 9 | 257 |
| Skiing, downhill (vigorous effort) | 11 | 343 |
| Sledding | 10 | 300 |
| Sleeping | 1 | 39 |
| Snowmobiling | 5 | 150 |
| Soccer (casual) | 10 | 300 |
| Softball or Baseball (fast or slow pitch) | 7 | 214 |
| Standing—playing with children (light) | 4 | 120 |
| Swimming (leisurely, not lap swimming) | 9 | 257 |
| Swimming Laps (freestyle, fast, vigorous effort) | 14 | 428 |
| Swimming Laps (freestyle, slow, moderate, or light effort | 11 | 343 |
| Tennis | 10 | 300 |
| Trampoline | 5 | 150 |
| Volleyball (non-competitive) | 4 | 129 |
| Walk/run—playing with children (moderate) | 6 | 171 |
| Walk/run—playing with children (vigorous) | 7 | 214 |
| Walking (carrying infant or 15-lb. load) | 5 | 150 |
| Walking (pushing a stroller with child) | 4 | 107 |
| Walking, 2.0 mph (level, slow pace, firm surface) | 4 | 107 |

| AEROBIC EXERCISE: CALORIE EXPENDITURE CHART | | |
|---|---|---|
| Activity | Calories burned per minute | Calories burned in 30 minutes |
| Walking, 3.0 mph (level, moderate pace, firm surface) | 5 | 150 |
| Walking, 4.0 mph (level, firm surface, very brisk pace) | 6 | 171 |
| Walking for Pleasure (walking the dog, work break) | 5 | 150 |
| Walking Shopping | 3 | 99 |
| Washing dishes (standing) | 3 | 99 |
| Water Aerobics | 6 | 171 |
| Watering Lawn or Garden (standing or walking) | 2 | 64 |
| Weight Lifting (light to moderate effort) | 4 | 129 |

*Source: MET to kilocalorie estimations derived from ACSMs Guidelines for Exercise Testing and Prescription, 6th Ed. 2000, Lippincott Williams & Wilkins, Baltimore, p. 308. MET value estimations based on 180-pound derived from ACSMs Resource Manual for Guidelines foe Exercise Testing and Prescription. Third Edition. Copyright 1998, pages 656–665.*

The purpose of this chart is to help you understand how many calories are burned for specific activities. The numbers in this chart are accurate for a 180-pound person—if you weigh more, you'll burn more calories per minute; if you weigh less, you'll burn less.

## Action 3: Strength Training

In order to accomplish your 30-minutes of strength training at least two days per week, you can use the workout described in this book, hire a personal trainer, or create your own strength-training workout. Beginning on page 162, there is a home workout using an exercise ball and resistance tubing or hand weights. The program specifies a "weekly workout," such as "Week 1," "Week 2," and so forth. Each week, the workouts change slightly to keep your body challenged and avoid boredom. Regardless of which method you choose to use, remember to keep the basics of strength training in mind:

- Sets: Two to three per exercise.

- Repetitions: 8 to 15.

- Intensity: Resistance should be heavy enough that the last two to three reps are extremely challenging.

- Frequency: Two to three days per week, on alternating days.

# Action 4: Commit

There are two important factors that will play into your personal success with a new exercise program: (1) what you *should* do, and (2) what you *can* do. By now, you know what you should do in order to improve health and manage weight successfully:

1. Engage in 30 to 90 minutes of aerobic activity five to six days per week.
2. Complete 6 to 10 strength-training exercises (30 to 45 minutes) two to three days per week.
3. Follow your meal plan until you learn how to choose wisely for yourself.

That sounds simple, but realistically, does a program like this fit into your busy life? This is the reason for factor 2: *What you can do.* It is perfectly okay to admit that taking on too much at one time can be overwhelming, and even more important, can be unrealistic and non-maintainable. I want you to start something you enjoy—something you can stick with for the rest of your life. Therefore, even though you may not lose weight as fast, or see the benefits as quickly as others, if you need to start with two days per week, then great—go for it! At least you are taking a giant step in the right direction. I have always believed, and continue to believe, that if you can simply *start* exercising—one or two days a week—you will feel the invigorating, uplifting effects of exercise, and you will *want* to do more exercise with each passing day.

So let's start thinking about your personal workout program. Keep in mind that if you want to lose one to two pounds per week (which is healthy and maintainable!), then you need to create a calorie deficit of 3,500 (one pound) to 7,000 (two pounds) calories per week, or 500 to 1,000 calories per day. You can do this by setting a goal to burn 250 to 500 calories per workout and by cutting 250 to 500 calories from your daily food intake. Now, let's get you started. The first step is to commit—take a moment to evaluate your typical day and decide what will work for you:

- I will work out in the (morning/afternoon/evening).
- I will work out (2/3/4/5/6) days per week.
- I can fit a (30/60/90)-minute workout into my day.

I have worked in the fitness industry since I was 18 years old. Through my experiences as a group-fitness program director, personal trainer, consulting dietitian, and mother who struggles every day to squeeze in a workout, I feel that I have seen and heard it all. Really, I have learned two important things: (1) get your workouts done at the first of the week, and (2) get your workouts done in the morning. In the past eleven years, I have always seen a clear pattern on Thursday, Friday, and Saturday: these were always the days that my clients were more likely to not show up. These were the days on which the group fitness classes had lower attendance and when families seemed to be busy with weekend commitments, household duties, or other events. Therefore, if it seems that the following sample workout schedules are heavily weighted toward the first part of the week—they are. You have already made the first step to commit. What did you commit to? Thirty minutes? For five days per week? Whatever it was, read through the chart on page 136 to find the schedule that will work best with *your* schedule.

Regardless of which program you decide will work with your schedule, it is important to pick one and just get started! It is also important to commit to the program for at least eight weeks—you really need this amount of time on a structured program to help you establish new habits. In fact, eight weeks is quite short. However, I want this to be a realistic goal, and I truly believe that eight weeks is short enough to allow you to see a light at the end of the tunnel but long enough to learn the foundations of healthy eating and exercise. Following a disciplined program for a short time is essential to help you get through that "fight or flight" stage, in which you aren't sure if your efforts are really worth it. However, you are not off the hook after following the program for eight weeks. Rather, after eight weeks you will have the knowledge and experience you need to make healthy choices on your own. You will know what to do, and you simply need to take action—for yourself and your health! Some people may choose to repeat the eight-week commitment to the program, which is absolutely fine. If you do well with structure, then go for it. In fact, in eight weeks, you may not be at your dream weight (losing 25 pounds healthfully will take a good 12 weeks), but you will have the self-reliance and self-confidence to know that you are making the right decisions for your health. Most important, you will have the self-reliance to stick with a program that fits into the fast-paced action of real life.

| COMMITMENT LEVEL: 30-MINUTE WORKOUT 2 DAYS PER WEEK | | | | | |
|---|---|---|---|---|---|
| **Monday** | **Tuesday** | **Wednesday** | **Thursday** | **Friday** | **Saturday** |
| Cardio | | Cardio | | | |

| COMMITMENT LEVEL: 30-MINUTE WORKOUT 3 DAYS PER WEEK | | | | | |
|---|---|---|---|---|---|
| **Monday** | **Tuesday** | **Wednesday** | **Thursday** | **Friday** | **Saturday** |
| Cardio | | Cardio | | Cardio | |

| COMMITMENT LEVEL: 30-MINUTE WORKOUT 4 DAYS PER WEEK | | | | | |
|---|---|---|---|---|---|
| **Monday** | **Tuesday** | **Wednesday** | **Thursday** | **Friday** | **Saturday** |
| Cardio | Strength | Cardio | | Strength | |

| COMMITMENT LEVEL: 30-MINUTE WORKOUT 5 DAYS PER WEEK | | | | | |
|---|---|---|---|---|---|
| **Monday** | **Tuesday** | **Wednesday** | **Thursday** | **Friday** | **Saturday** |
| Cardio | Strength | Cardio | Strength | Cardio | |

| COMMITMENT LEVEL: 30-MINUTE WORKOUT 6 DAYS PER WEEK | | | | | |
|---|---|---|---|---|---|
| **Monday** | **Tuesday** | **Wednesday** | **Thursday** | **Friday** | **Saturday** |
| Cardio | Strength | Cardio | Strength | Cardio | Strength or Cardio |

| COMMITMENT LEVEL: 60-MINUTE WORKOUT 2 DAYS PER WEEK | | | | | |
|---|---|---|---|---|---|
| **Monday** | **Tuesday** | **Wednesday** | **Thursday** | **Friday** | **Saturday** |
| 30 min Cardio & 30 min Strength | | 30 min Cardio & 30 min Strength | | | |

| COMMITMENT LEVEL: 60-MINUTE WORKOUT 3 DAYS PER WEEK | | | | | |
|---|---|---|---|---|---|
| **Monday** | **Tuesday** | **Wednesday** | **Thursday** | **Friday** | **Saturday** |
| 30 min Cardio & 30 min Strength | | 30 min Cardio & 30 min Strength | | 30 min Cardio & 30 min Strength | |

| COMMITMENT LEVEL: 60-MINUTE WORKOUT 4 DAYS PER WEEK | | | | | |
|---|---|---|---|---|---|
| **Monday** | **Tuesday** | **Wednesday** | **Thursday** | **Friday** | **Saturday** |
| 30 min Cardio & 30 min Strength | 60 min Cardio | 30 min Cardio & 30 min Strength | | 30 min Cardio & 30 min Strength | |

| COMMITMENT LEVEL: 60–90-MINUTE WORKOUT 5 DAYS PER WEEK | | | | | |
|---|---|---|---|---|---|
| **Monday** | **Tuesday** | **Wednesday** | **Thursday** | **Friday** | **Saturday** |
| 30-45 min Cardio & 30 min Strength (upper body) | 30-45 min Cardio & 30 min Strength (lower body) | 30-45 min Cardio & 30 min Strength (upper body) | 30-45 min Cardio & 30 min Strength (lower body) | | 30-45 min Strength (total body workout) & 30 min Cardio |

| COMMITMENT LEVEL: 60–90-MINUTE WORKOUT 6 DAYS PER WEEK | | | | | |
|---|---|---|---|---|---|
| **Monday** | **Tuesday** | **Wednesday** | **Thursday** | **Friday** | **Saturday** |
| Cardio | Strength | Cardio | Strength | Cardio | Strength or Cardio |

# The Flexible Meal Planner

| BREAKFAST<br>All breakfast options are about 400 calories | |
|---|---|
| **Option 1** | **Calories** |
| 1 ½ cups whole-grain cereal with 3 or more grams of fiber | 180 |
| 1 cup 1% low-fat or skim milk | 110 |
| 1 banana | 110 |
| **Total** | 400 |
| **Option 2** | **Calories** |
| 2 slices whole-wheat toast | 200 |
| 1 tsp. canola spread | 30 |
| 1 Tbsp. jam | 60 |
| 1 cup orange juice with calcium | 110 |
| **Total** | 400 |
| **Option 3** | **Calories** |
| ½ cup dry oatmeal (prepare with water) | 155 |
| 1 tsp. brown sugar | 15 |
| 2 tsp. ground flaxseed | 30 |
| 2 scrambled eggs (use 2 egg whites to 1 yolk) | 100 |
| 1 cup orange juice with calcium | 110 |
| **Total** | 410 |
| **Option 4** | **Calories** |
| 8 oz. plain yogurt | 165 |
| 1 cup sliced strawberries | 50 |
| 1 slice whole-wheat toast | 100 |
| 1 Tbsp. natural peanut butter | 95 |
| Water | 0 |
| **Total** | 410 |
| **Option 5** | **Calories** |
| 1 cup low-fat cottage cheese | 160 |
| 2 cups melon or fresh fruit | 100 |
| ½ whole-wheat bagel | 100 |
| 2 tsp. jam | 40 |
| Water | 0 |
| **Total** | 400 |

# BREAKFAST CONTINUED
## All breakfast options are about 400 calories

| Option 6 | Calories |
|---|---|
| 1 hard-boiled egg | 78 |
| 1 whole-wheat english muffin | 130 |
| 1 Tbsp. jam mixed with 1 tsp. ground flaxseed | 75 |
| 1 cup 1% low-fat milk or orange juice with calcium | 110 |
| Water | 0 |
| **Total** | 393 |
| **Option 7** | **Calories** |
| Spinach and Cheese Omelette: | |
|    1 whole egg and 1 egg white | 100 |
|    ¼ cup spinach | 15 |
|    ¼ cup reduced-fat cheese | 90 |
| 1 cup fresh berries | 80 |
| 1 cup 1% low-fat or skim milk | 110 |
| **Total** | 395 |
| **Option 8** | **Calories** |
| 2 NutriGrain® Frozen Waffles | 142 |
| 2 tsp. canola spread | 60 |
| 2 Tbsp. maple syrup | 100 |
| 1 cup 1% low-fat or skim milk | 110 |
| **Total** | 412 |
| **Option 9** | **Calories** |
| Breakfast Wrap: | |
|    1 whole-wheat tortilla | 140 |
|    2 scrambled eggs (use 2 egg whites to 1 yolk) | 100 |
|    ¼ cup reduced-fat cheese | 90 |
|    2 Tbsp. salsa | 10 |
| 1 medium fresh fruit | 80 |
| Water | 0 |
| **Total** | 420 |

# BREAKFAST CONTINUED
## All breakfast options are about 400 calories

| Option 10—On the Go | Calories |
|---|---|
| 1 small (16–20 oz.) fruit smoothie | 400 |
| with added flaxseed | 0 |
| Water | 0 |
| **Total** | 400 |
| **Option 11—On the Go** | **Calories** |
| McDonald's® Fruit and Yogurt Parfait with Granola (small 5 oz.) | 160 |
| 2 scrambled eggs (side order) | 160 |
| Water | 0 |
| **Total** | 320 |
| **Option 12—On the Go** | **Calories** |
| Crossan'wich® with Egg and Cheese (300 calories) -OR- McDonalds® Egg McMuffin (300 calories) | |
| or- Einstein Bros® Honey Whole Wheat Bagel w/2 Tbsp. cream cheese | 390 |
| Water | 0 |
| **Total** | 390 |
| **Option 13—On the Go** | **Calories** |
| Best "Dine in" Restaurant Breakfast: | |
| Hot or cold cereal with low-fat milk | 210 |
| Scrambled egg substitute | 130 |
| 1/2 cup fresh fruit | 50 |
| **Total** | 390 |
| **Option 14—On the Go** | **Calories** |
| 1 medium low-fat bran muffin** | 300 |
| 1 medium fresh fruit | 80 |
| Water | 0 |
| **Total** | 380 |

**Try to skip huge muffins, scones, pastries, and monster cinnamon rolls or only enjoy a ½ portion at a time.*

# BREAKFAST CONTINUED
## All breakfast options are about 400 calories

| Option 15 | Calories |
|---|---|
| 2 slices french toast (homemade using 2 slices whole-grain bread, skim milk, 1 egg, and cinnamon and vanilla) | 260 |
| 2 Tbsp. maple syrup | 100 |
| ½ cup berries | 40 |
| Water | 0 |
| **Total** | 400 |
| **Option 16** | **Calories** |
| ½ cup low-fat cottage cheese with 1 Tbsp. ground flaxseed and ½ cup sliced strawberries | 160 |
| 1 hard-boiled egg | 80 |
| 1 cup orange juice with calcium | 110 |
| **Total** | 350 |
| **Option 17** | **Calories** |
| Yogurt Mixer: | |
| 6 oz. light yogurt | 100 |
| ½ cup GrapeNuts® or other high-fiber cereal | 200 |
| 1 cup berries (fresh or frozen) | 80 |
| Water | 0 |
| **Total** | 380 |
| **Option 18** | **Calories** |
| 2 whole-wheat pancakes (4" each) | 184 |
| 1 tsp. canola spread | 30 |
| 2 Tbsp. maple syrup | 100 |
| 2 scrambled eggs (use 2 egg whites to 1 yolk) | 100 |
| Water | 0 |
| **Total** | 414 |
| **Option 19** | **Calories** |
| 1 NutriGrain® cereal bar | 140 |
| 1 oz. almonds | 180 |
| 1½ cup melon | 75 |
| **Total** | 395 |

## BREAKFAST CONTINUED
### All breakfast options are about 400 calories

| Option 20 | Calories |
|---|---|
| 1¾ cups whole-grain cereal with 3 or more grams of fiber | 210 |
| 1 medium fruit or 1 cup berries | 80 |
| 1 cup 1% low-fat milk or orange juice with calcium | 110 |
| Total | 400 |

| Option 21 | Calories |
|---|---|
| Breakfast Sandwich: | |
| 1 whole-wheat english muffin | 130 |
| 2 scrambled eggs (use 2 egg whites to 1 yolk) | 100 |
| 2 slices canadian bacon | 87 |
| 1 cup orange juice with calcium | 110 |
| Total | 427 |

## LUNCH
### All lunch options are 400 calories

| Option 1 | Calories |
|---|---|
| Deli Sandwich: | 305 |
| 2 slices whole-wheat bread | |
| 2 oz. lean deli meat | |
| 2 tsp. light mayonnaise | |
| 1 tsp. yellow mustard | |
| vegetables of choice | |
| 1 medium fruit | 80 |
| Water | 0 |
| Total | 385 |

| Option 2 | Calories |
|---|---|
| Pita Sandwich: | 385 |
| 1 whole-wheat pita (6½'') | |
| 2 oz. lean deli meat | |
| 1 oz. cheese | |
| 2 tsp. light mayonnaise | |
| 1 tsp. yellow mustard | |
| vegetables of choice | |

## LUNCH CONTINUED
### All lunch options are about 400 calories

| Option 2 continued... | Calories |
|---|---|
| 5–7 baby carrots | 23 |
| Water | 0 |
| Total | 408 |
| **Option 3** | **Calories** |
| 1 ½ cups broth-based or bean soup (preferably low-sodium) | 150 |
| 1 slice cheese toast: | 206 |
|    1 slice whole-wheat toast | |
|    1 oz. slice cheese | |
| ½ cup grapes or other fresh fruit | 57 |
| Water | 0 |
| Total | 413 |
| **Option 4** | **Calories** |
| Chicken-Breast Salad: | 290 |
|    1 grilled or baked chicken breast (no breading) | |
|    4 cups tossed greens with vegetables | |
|    ¼ cup low-fat salad dressing | |
|    1 whole-wheat dinner roll | 100 |
| Water | 0 |
| Total | 390 |
| **Option 5** | **Calories** |
| Tuna Sandwich: | 355 |
|    2 slices whole-wheat bread | |
|    ½ can (or 3 oz.) tuna in spring water | |
|    1 Tbsp. light mayonnaise | |
|    ½ oz. baked chips (about 6 chips) | 60 |
| Water | 0 |
| Total | 415 |
| **Option 6** | **Calories** |
| Peanut Butter and Jam Sandwich: | 403 |
|    2 slices whole-wheat bread | |
|    1 Tbsp. natural peanut butter | |
|    1 Tbsp. jam | |

# LUNCH CONTINUED
## All lunch options are about 400 calories

| Option 6 continued... | Calories |
|---|---|
| 5–7 baby carrots | 23 |
| ½ cup cubed melon or ¼ cup fresh fruit | 30 |
| Water | 0 |
| **Total** | 403 |
| **Option 7** | **Calories** |
| ½ sandwich on whole-wheat bread (choose from the following): | 175 |
|     deli, tuna, or peanut butter and jam | |
| 2 cups tossed greens with vegetables | 25 |
| 2 Tbsp. low-fat or fat-free salad dressing | 50 |
| 1 medium fruit | 80 |
| ½ oz. baked chips (about 6 chips) | 60 |
| Water | 0 |
| **Total** | 390 |
| **Option 8—On the Go** | **Calories** |
| Lean Cuisine® or Healthy Choice® frozen entrée   400 calories | 400 |
| Water | 0 |
| **Total** | 400 |
| **Option 9—On the Go** | **Calories** |
| Subway® or 6" sub on wheat bread with vegetables: | 300 |
|     Choose from  ham, turkey, turkey and ham, roast beef, veggie | |
|     no cheese or mayonnaise | |
|     light vinegar, mustard | |
| 1 oz. baked chips (one small bag) | 120 |
| Water | 0 |
| **Total** | 420 |

## LUNCH CONTINUED
### All lunch options are about 400 calories

| Option 10—On the Go | Calories |
|---|---|
| 1 grilled chicken sandwich without mayonnaise (from a fast-food or dine-in restaurant) | 300 |
| 1 side salad | 75 |
| 2 Tbsp. low-fat salad dressing | 50 |
| Water | 0 |
| **Total** | 425 |
| **Option 11—On the Go** | **Calories** |
| 1 large or 2 small soft chicken tacos | 430 |
| Water | 0 |
| **Total** | 430 |
| **Option 12—On the Go** | **Calories** |
| Panda Express® (choose 2 of the following): | 400 |
| Black Pepper Chicken | |
| Chicken with Mushrooms | |
| Chicken with String Beans | |
| Spicy Chicken with Peanuts | |
| Beef with Broccoli | |
| Beef with String Beans | |
| Vegetable Chow Mein (1⁄2 order) | |
| Steamed Rice (1⁄2 order) | |
| Water | 0 |
| **Total** | 400 |
| **Option 13—On the Go** | **Calories** |
| McDonald's® Salad (choose 1 of the following): | 400 |
| Grilled Chicken Bacon Ranch Salad with 3⁄4 packet Newman's Own® Ranch dressing | |
| Grilled Chicken Caesar Salad with 1 packet Newman's Own® Creamy Caesar Dressing | |
| Grilled Chicken California Cobb Salad with 1 packet Newman's Own® Cobb Dressing | |

| LUNCH CONTINUED<br>All lunch options are about 400 calories | |
|---|---|
| **Option 13—On the Go continued...** | **Calories** |
| Fruit and Walnut Salad | |
| Water | 0 |
| **Total** | 310 |
| **Option 14—On the Go** | **Calories** |
| Burger King® Salad (choose 1 of the following): | 400 |
| Fire-Grilled Caesar Salad<br>(chicken or shrimp) with 1 packet dressing and 1 slice garlic parmesan toast | |
| Fire-Grilled Garden Salad<br>(chicken or shrimp) with 1 packet dressing and 1 slice garlic parmesan toast | |
| Water | 0 |
| **Total** | 400 |
| **Option 15—On the Go** | **Calories** |
| Wendy's® Salad (choose 1 of the following): | 400 |
| Spring Mix Salad with pecans and ½ packet House Vinaigrette Dressing | |
| Mandarin Chicken® Salad<br>with almonds and ½ packet Oriental Sesame Dressing | |
| Water | 0 |
| **Total** | 400 |
| **Option 16—On the Go** | **Calories** |
| Arby's® Salad (choose 1 of the following): | 400 |
| Martha's Vineyard™ Salad<br>with almonds and ½ packet Raspberry Vinaigrette Dressing | |
| Asian Sesame™ Salad<br>with almonds, Asian noodles, and ½ packet Asian Sesame Dressing | |
| Water | 0 |
| **Total** | 400 |
| **Option 17—On the Go** | **Calories** |
| Schlotsky's Deli®: | 400 |
| 1 small Chicken Breast or Smoked Turkey Hot Sandwich | |
| 1 small piece fresh fruit | |
| Water | 0 |
| **Total** | 400 |

## LUNCH CONTINUED
### All lunch options are about 400 calories

| Option 17—On the Go continued... | Calories |
|---|---|
| Sbarro®: | 400 |
|    1 slice Low-Carb Cheese Pizza | |
|    1 (8-oz.) Mixed Garden Salad w/low-fat dressing | |
| Water | 0 |
| TacoMaker®: | 400 |
|    1 Chicken Burrito OR 1 Super Soft Taco | |
| Water | 0 |
| **Total** | 400 |
| **Option 18** | **Calories** |
| 1 ½ cups whole-wheat spaghetti | 260 |
| ½ cup pasta sauce | 90 |
| 1 medium fruit | 80 |
| Water | 0 |
| **Total** | 430 |
| **Option 19** | **Calories** |
| 1 ½ cups broth-based soup or 1 cup chili | 200 |
| 2 cups tossed greens with vegetables | 25 |
| 2 Tbsp. low-fat salad dressing | 50 |
| 1 whole-wheat breadstick | 100 |
| Water | 0 |
| **Total** | 375 |
| **Option 20—On the Go** | **Calories** |
| Olive Garden®: | |
|    1 order Minestrone soup | 164 |
|    1 serving salad (estimated from USDA website and salad dressing label) | 125 |
|    1 breadstick | 140 |
| Water | 0 |
| **Total** | 429 |
| **Option 21—On the Go** | **Calories** |
| ½ order (about 2 ½ cups) stir-fried vegetables with steamed rice | 400 |
| Water | 0 |

# DINNER
## All dinner options are about 500 calories

| Option 1—Gourmet | Calories |
|---|---|
| 4 oz. Steamed Salmon with Black Bean Sauce | 240 |
| 1 cup vegetables, steamed<br>(i.e. asparagus, broccoli, cauliflower, green beans, summer squash, zucchini) | 50 |
| 1 whole-wheat dinner roll | 90 |
| 1 tsp. canola spread | 40 |
| 1 cup 1% low-fat or skim milk | 110 |
| Water | 0 |
| **Total** | 530 |

| Option 2—Gourmet | Calories |
|---|---|
| 4 oz. Creole Pork Tenderloin | 231 |
| ⅓ cup Apple Jicama Salsa | 45 |
| ½ cup vegetables, steamed (asparagus, broccoli, cauliflower, green beans) | 25 |
| ½ cup boiled red potatoes | 70 |
| 1 tsp. canola spread | 40 |
| 1 cup 1% low-fat or skim milk | 110 |
| Water | 0 |
| **Total** | 521 |

| Option 3—Gourmet | Calories |
|---|---|
| 1 Chicken Enchilada with salsa and 1 Tbsp. light sour cream | 290 |
| 2 cups tossed greens with vegetables | 25 |
| 2 Tbsp. low-fat salad dressing | 50 |
| ½ cup cubed melon | 30 |
| 1 cup 1% low-fat or skim milk | 110 |
| Water | 0 |
| **Total** | 505 |

| Option 4—Quick & Easy | Calories |
|---|---|
| 1 Marinated Chicken Breast | 170 |
| 1 medium baked sweet potato | 117 |
| 1 tsp. canola spread | 40 |
| 1 tsp. brown sugar | 15 |
| 2 cups tossed greens with vegetables | 25 |

# DINNER CONTINUED
## All dinner options are about 500 calories

| Option 4—Quick & Easy continued... | Calories |
|---|---|
| 2 Tbsp. low-fat salad dressing | 50 |
| 1 cup 1% low-fat or skim milk | 110 |
| Water | 0 |
| **Total** | 527 |
| **Option 5—Gourmet** | **Calories** |
| 1 cup Roasted Tomato Pasta | 335 |
| 2 cups tossed greens with vegetables | 25 |
| 2 Tbsp. low-fat or fat-free salad dressing | 50 |
| 1 cup 1% low-fat or skim milk | 110 |
| Water | 0 |
| **Total** | 520 |
| **Option 6—On the Go** | **Calories** |
| Chinese restaurant, ½ entrée order with rice (choose 1 of the following): | 500 |
| Szechwan shrimp | |
| Shrimp with garlic sauce | |
| Beef with broccoli | |
| Chicken chow mein | |
| Water | 0 |
| **Total** | 500 |
| **Option 7—On the Go** | **Calories** |
| Chili's® Guiltless Chicken Sandwich | 528 |
| (or grilled chicken breast sandwich with no-fat honey mustard; black beans; steamed vegetables) | |
| Water | 0 |
| **Total** | 528 |
| **Option 8—On the Go** | **Calories** |
| Grilled chicken breast (barbecue or other seasoning) | 270 |
| House salad with 2 Tbsp. light or fat-free dressing | 150 |
| ½ baked potato with salt and pepper | 100 |
| Water | 0 |
| **Total** | 520 |

# DINNER CONTINUED
## All dinner options are about 500 calories

| Option 9—On the Go | Calories |
|---|---|
| 2 slices Domino's Pizza® Classic Hand Tossed medium pizza (choose from the following pizzas/toppings): | 450 |
| Deluxe Feast; Vegi Feast; Hawaiian Feast | |
| Choose own toppings: Canadian bacon and/or any vegetables | |
| 2 cups tossed greens with vegetables | 25 |
| 2 Tbsp. low-fat or fat-free salad dressing | 50 |
| Water | 0 |
| **Total** | 525 |

| Option 10—Quick & Easy | Calories |
|---|---|
| 1½ cups stir-fry with chicken or shrimp | 230 |
| ½ cup brown rice | 108 |
| ½cup mixed fresh fruit | 50 |
| 1 cup 1% low-fat or skim milk | 110 |
| Water | 0 |
| **Total** | 498 |

| Option 11—Quick & Easy | Calories |
|---|---|
| 6 oz. lemon halibut | 243 |
| ½ cup wild rice mix | 100 |
| ½ cup vegetables, steamed | 25 |
| 1 cup berries or melons | 50 |
| 1 cup 1% low-fat or skim milk | 110 |
| Water | 0 |
| **Total** | 528 |

| Option 12—Quick & Easy | Calories |
|---|---|
| 1 cup whole-wheat spaghetti | 175 |
| ½cup spaghetti sauce with lean ground beef | 140 |
| 2 cups tossed greens with vegetables | 25 |
| 2 Tbsp. low-fat or fat-free salad dressing | 50 |
| 1 cup 1% low-fat or skim milk | 110 |
| Water | 0 |
| **Total** | 500 |

## DINNER CONTINUED
### All dinner options are about 500 calories

| Option 13—Quick & Easy | Calories |
|---|---|
| 1 french dip sandwich | 333 |
| 2 cups tossed greens with vegetables | 25 |
| 2 Tbsp. low-fat salad dressing | 50 |
| ¾ cup mixed fresh fruit | 75 |
| Water | 0 |
| **Total** | 483 |
| **Option 14—Quick & Easy** | **Calories** |
| 4 oz. sirloin steak (from 6 oz. raw) or 1 (3-oz.) lean hamburger patty | 240 |
| ½ cup boiled red potatoes | 67 |
| 1 tsp. canola spread | 40 |
| 1 cup vegetables, steamed (i.e. asparagus, broccoli, cauliflower, green beans, summer squash, zucchini) | 50 |
| 1 whole wheat dinner roll | 90 |
| Water | 0 |
| **Total** | 487 |
| **Option 15—Quick & Easy** | **Calories** |
| 4 oz. marinated turkey tenderloin | 170 |
| ½ cup rice pilaf | 130 |
| ½ cup green peas | 60 |
| 1 cup 1% low-fat or skim milk | 110 |
| Water | 0 |
| **Total** | 470 |
| **Option 16—Gourmet** | **Calories** |
| 1 ½ cups Chicken Divan Casserole | 350 |
| 2 cups tossed greens with vegetables | 25 |
| 2 Tbsp. low-fat salad dressing | 50 |
| ¾ cup mixed fresh fruit | 75 |
| Water | 0 |
| **Total** | 500 |

# DINNER CONTINUED
## All dinner options are about 500 calories

| Option 17—Gourmet | Calories |
|---|---|
| 4 oz. Fish Fillet with Orange-Rosemary Sauce | 198 |
| ½ small baked potato (top with 1 Tbsp. light sour cream and sprinkle with powdered ranch dressing mix) | 120 |
| ½ cup vegetables, steamed (i.e. asparagus, broccoli, cauliflower, green beans, summer squash, zucchini) | 25 |
| ¾ cup mixed fresh fruit | 75 |
| 1 cup 1% low-fat or skim milk | 110 |
| Water | 0 |
| **Total** | 528 |

| Option 18—Quick & Easy | Calories |
|---|---|
| 1 ½ cups chili | 340 |
| 1 whole-wheat dinner roll or breadstick | 90 |
| 1 cup raw vegetables (i.e. carrots, celery, broccoli, cucumbers, and cherry tomatoes) | 40 |
| 2 Tbsp. low-fat salad dressing | 50 |
| Water | 0 |
| **Total** | 520 |

| Option 19—Gourmet | Calories |
|---|---|
| 1 Steak Fajita with salsa | 315 |
| ½ Tbsp. guacamole | 32 |
| ⅓ cup Spicy Black Beans | 75 |
| ¾ cup mixed fresh fruit | 75 |
| Water | 0 |
| **Total** | 497 |

| Option 20—Gourmet | Calories |
|---|---|
| Mediterranean Pesto Chicken (1 breast) | 275 |
| ¾ cup whole-wheat pasta | 130 |
| ½ cup vegetables, steamed (i.e. asparagus, broccoli, cauliflower, green beans, summer squash, zucchini) | 25 |
| 1 cup 1% low-fat or skim milk | 110 |
| Water | 0 |
| **Total** | 540 |

## DINNER CONTINUED
### All dinner options are about 500 calories

| Option 21–Quick & Easy | Calories |
|---|---|
| Taco Salad: | |
| 10 baked tortilla chips | 85 |
| ¾ cup extra lean ground beef with taco seasoning | 135 |
| ½ cup refried beans | 120 |
| 2 Tbsp. shredded reduced-fat cheese | 25 |
| 2 Tbsp. sliced olives | 20 |
| 2 cups tossed greens with vegetables | 25 |
| 3 Tbsp. light sour cream | 50 |
| ¼ cup salsa | 15 |
| ½ cup mixed fresh fruit | 50 |
| Water | 0 |
| **Total** | 525 |

# VEGETABLES
## All good options — Choose best option for your calorie budget

| FOOD | KCAL | FOOD | KCAL |
|---|---|---|---|
| ½ cup mushrooms (raw or cooked) | 12 | 1 cup cooked green beans | 44 |
| ½ cucumber, sliced | 14 | 1 cup mixed vegetables | 50 |
| 1½ cup leafy greens | 15 | 1 cup cooked okra | 50 |
| 1 cup shredded cabbage | 17 | 1 cup vegetable juice | 53 |
| 1 cup sliced sweet peppers | 18 | ½ cup boiled potatoes | 57 |
| 1 cup sliced zucchini | 18 | ½ medium sweet potato | 58 |
| 1 cup broccoli (raw or cooked) | 20 | ½ cup green peas | 64 |
| 1 cup cooked asparagus (6 spears) | 20 | ½ cup corn | 66 |
| 2 cups chopped collards, spinach or swiss chard | 20 | 1 cup sugar snap peas | 75 |
| 1 cup cherry tomatoes or 1 medium tomato | 25 | 1 cup colesslaw | 82 |
| 1 cup raw cauliflower | 25 | corn on the cob | 83 |
| 5 fava beans in pod | 18 | ½ medium baked potato | 100 |
| 1 cucumber | 28 | ⅓ cup canned kidney beans | 113 |
| ½ cup brussel sprouts | 28 | ½ cup canned black beans | 114 |
| 3 cups leafy greens | 30 | ½ cup cooked lentils | 115 |
| 8 (4") celery sticks | 32 | 1 medium sweet potato | 116 |
| 1 cup kale | 34 | ½ cup baked beans | 120 |
| 1 cup baby carrots (about 15 each) | 35 | ½ cup mashed potatoes | 122 |
| 1 cup cooked summer squash | 36 | ½ cup cooked soybeans | 127 |

## FRUITS
### All good options – Choose best option for your calorie budget

| FOOD | KCAL | FOOD | KCAL |
|---|---|---|---|
| 1 apricot | 17 | 1 cup fresh berries | 60 |
| 1 date | 23 | ½ papaya | 60 |
| ½ cup sliced strawberries | 23 | 2 plums | 60 |
| 2 small kumquats | 26 | 1 cup diced honeydew | 61 |
| ½ cup cubed cantaloupe | 27 | ⅛ cup raisins | 62 |
| ½ cup cubed melons | 30 | 1 orange | 65 |
| 1 plum | 30 | 3 dates | 66 |
| ½ cup fresh berries | 32 | 1 cup canned pears | 70 |
| 1 persimmon | 32 | 1 cup fresh pineapple | 74 |
| ½ cup canned pears | 35 | 1 grapefruit | 74 |
| ½ cup fresh pineapple | 35 | 1 apple | 81 |
| 1 peach | 38 | 1 cup blueberries/mixed berries | 83 |
| ½ cup canned pineapple | 40 | ¾ cup orange juice | 84 |
| ½ cup cherries | 45 | ¾ cup cranberry juice | 87 |
| 1 cup watermelon | 46 | 1 cup raw cherries | 90 |
| 1 kiwi fruit | 46 | 1 pear | 96 |
| ½ grapefruit | 48 | ¼ cup dried fruit (small handful) | 100 |
| 3 apricots | 51 | 1 cup unsweetened applesauce | 105 |
| ½ cup mandarin oranges/juice | 51 | 1 pomegranate | 105 |
| ½ medium banana | 51 | 1 banana | 110 |
| ½ cup unsweetened applesauce | 52 | 1 cup red/green grapes | 110 |
| 1 cup cubed cantaloupe | 54 | 1 cup orange juice | 112 |
| ½ cup red/green grapes | 55 | ½ cup sliced avocado | 116 |
| ½ cup cranberry juice | 58 | 1 medium papaya fruit | 120 |
| ¼ cup sliced avocado | 58 | ¼ cup raisins | 124 |
| | | 1 cup sliced mango | 130 |

| HEALTHY SNACKS | | | | | |
|---|---|---|---|---|---|
| **CHOOSE OFTEN** | | **CHOOSE CAUTIOUSLY** | | **USE SPARINGLY** | |
| FOOD | KCAL | FOOD | KCAL | FOOD | KCAL |
| 1 cup sugar free gelatin | 16 | ½ cup fat-free pudding | 100 | ⅓ cup granola | 200 |
| ½ cup non-fat frozen yogurt | 47 | 1 cup sherbet | 102 | 2 oatmeal raisin cookies | 212 |
| 15 baby carrots | 35 | 1 oz. whole-wheat pretzels | 110 | 1 cup TCBY® non-fat frozen yogurt | 220 |
| 1 Tbsp. sunflower seed kernels | 56 | 4 gingersnap cookies | 116 | 16 oz. Orange or Strawberry Original Orange Julius® | 220 |
| 2 cups popcorn | 60 | 1 cup dry whole-grain cereal | 120 | 2 oz. baked tortilla chips (approx. 20) | 220 |
| ½ cup dry whole-grain cereal | 60 | 1 low-fat granola bar | 125 | ⅓ cup trail mix | 233 |
| 4 whole-wheat crackers | 71 | ½ cup low-fat cottage cheese w/ ½ cup fruit | 150 | 20 oz. TCBY® Raspberry DeLITE Smoothie (w/o yogurt) | 240 |
| 1 frozen fruit bar | 75 | 1 cup plain low-fat yogurt | 160 | 15 whole-wheat crackers | 265 |
| 1 oz. string cheese | 80 | 1 whole-wheat english muffin w/ 2 tsp. Jam | 160 | | |
| 1 medium fresh fruit | 80 | 1 oz. almonds (small handful) | 170 | | |
| 1 cup melon or berries | 100 | 1 oz. walnuts | 180 | | |

| SNACKS ON THE GO | | | | | |
|---|---|---|---|---|---|
| **CHOOSE OFTEN** | | **CHOOSE CAUTIOUSLY** | | **USE SPARINGLY** | |
| **FOOD** | **KCAL** | **FOOD** | **KCAL** | **FOOD** | **KCAL** |
| 8 oz. vegetable juice | 50 | 1 cup low-fat milk | 110 | 1 small soft taco | 215 |
| 1 cup raw veggies (carrots, peppers, cucumbers, etc) | 50 | 1 oz. cheddar cheese | 110 | 20-oz. regular soda | 220 |
| Dairy Queen® Sugar-Free Fudge Bar | 60 | 1 oz. baked chips (about 12) | 110 | Mrs. Field's® Chocolate Chip cookie | 250 |
| 1 oz. string cheese (part-skim mozza-rella) | 80 | 1 oz. pretzel twists (about 20) | 110 | ½ cup ice cream | 250 |
| ½ cup low-fat cottage cheese | 80 | 1 cup soy milk | 120 | 1 donut | 250 |
| 1 medium piece fresh fruit | 80 | 1 (6-oz.) container non-fat yogurt | 120 | 1 large (12-oz.) chili | 310 |
| 1 oz. turkey jerky (1 large piece) | 80 | Granola bar | 125 | 1 ham (or turkey) and cheese sandwich on whole-wheat bread | 315 |
| ½ oz. nuts (about 10 nuts) | 90 | McDonald's® Vanilla Ice Cream Cone | 150 | 1 small cheeseburger | 360 |
| Mixed fruit cup/bowl | 100 | Small garden salad w/light salad dressing | 150 | 1 sour cream & chives baked potato | 370 |
| 1 cup vegetable or minestrone soup | 100 | McDonald's® Fruit and Yogurt Parfait (5 oz.) | 160 | 1 (20-oz.) fruit smoothie | 400 |

## COMBINATION FOODS

| CHOOSE OFTEN | | CHOOSE CAUTIOUSLY | | USE SPARINGLY | |
|---|---|---|---|---|---|
| FOOD | KCAL | FOOD | KCAL | FOOD | KCAL |
| 10 baked tortilla chips w/ 1/4 cup salsa | 100 | 1/2 cup brown rice w/ 1/2 cup fat-free refried beans | 208 | 1 cup spaghetti w/ meat | 300 |
| 1/2 baked potato w/ 1/4 cup salsa | 125 | 1 slice whole-wheat bread w/ 1 oz. cheese | 210 | 1 ham and cheese sandwich on whole-wheat bread | 315 |
| 1/2 cup raspberries w/ 2 Tbsp. non-fat sour cream, 2 Tbsp. chopped nuts and 1 tsp. Splenda® | 150 | 1 whole-wheat tortilla w/ 1 oz. cheddar cheese | 210 | 1 1/2 cups chef salad w/ 2 Tbsp. fat-free dressing | 315 |
| 1 small taco | 180 | 1 cup ravioli | 230 | 1 grilled cheese sandwich on whole-wheat bread | 320 |
| 1 slice thin crust cheese or vegetable pizza | 190 | 1 whole-wheat tortilla w/ 1/2 cup fat-free refried beans and 1/2 cup salsa | 230 | 1 bean and beef burrito | 320 |
| 1 slice whole-wheat bread w/ 1 Tbsp. natural peanut butter | 190 | 1 1/2 cups shrimp garden salad | 254 | 1 garden burger on whole-grain bun | 320 |
| | | 1 apple w/ 2 Tbsp. natural peanut butter | 260 | 6" sub sandwich on wheat | 350 |
| | | 1 cup low-fat yogurt w/ 1/4 cup granola | 290 | 1 single patty cheeseburger | 360 |
| | | | | 2 small tacos | 360 |
| | | | | 6 oz. Spinach quiche (1 slice) | 362 |
| | | | | 2 slices thin crust pizza | 380 |
| | | | | 1 broccoli and cheese potato | 400 |

| BAKED GOODS | | | | | |
|---|---|---|---|---|---|
| **CHOOSE OFTEN** | | **CHOOSE CAUTIOUSLY** | | **USE SPARINGLY** | |
| FOOD | KCAL | FOOD | KCAL | FOOD | KCAL |
| 1 slice multi-grain bread | 80 | 4 small gingersnap cookies | 120 | 1 piece of cake (2" square) | 264 |
| 1 slice raisin bread | 80 | 1 english muffin | 140 | 1 large muffin | 300 |
| 1 slice cinnamon swirl bread | 80 | 1 whole-wheat pita (6") | 170 | 1 piece of pie ($1/8$th of pie) | 300 |
| 1 dinner roll | 90 | 1 small muffin | 200 | Einstein Bros® Honey Whole Wheat Bagel (no cream cheese) | 320 |
| 1 small cookie (2" diameter) | 100 | 1 slice banana bread | 200 | $1/2$ large bakery sweet roll | 335 |
| 1 slice french bread | 100 | 1 piece carrot cake (2" square) | 200 | Einstein Bros® Honey Whole Wheat Bagel with 2 Tbsp. cream cheese | 390 |
| 1 slice garlic bread | 110 | 1 large cookie (3-4"diameter) | 250 | large frosted bakery brownie | 400 |

| PARTY SNACKS | | | | | |
|---|---|---|---|---|---|
| **CHOOSE OFTEN** | | **CHOOSE CAUTIOUSLY** | | **USE SPARINGLY** | |
| **FOOD** | **KCAL** | **FOOD** | **KCAL** | **FOOD** | **KCAL** |
| 1 small piece chocolate-covered bite-sized fruit | 53 | 1 small peanut butter cookie | 102 | Cheesecake (small sliver about 1/16) | 250 |
| 2 gingersnap cookies | 58 | 1 oatmeal raisin cookie | 106 | 1/4 cup bean dip with 1 oz. tortilla chips | 220 |
| 2 cups popcorn | 60 | 2 small pieces chocolate (or bite-size chocolate-covered fruit) | 106 | 1/3 cup trail mix | 233 |
| 1 slice raisin bread | 70 | 1 oz. pretzels (about 20 twists) | 110 | 2" square brownie | 240 |
| 1 chocolate chip cookie (2 1/4" diam.) | 78 | 1 oz. baked potato chips (about 12) | 110 | 8 crackers with 1 oz. cheese | 250 |
| 1/2 oz. nuts (~10 nuts) | 90 | 1 oz. tortilla chips (about 12) | 140 | 2 oz. chocolate cake (2" square) | 264 |
| 1/2 cup 3-bean salad | 90 | 1/4 cup fruit dip with 1/2 cup fresh fruit | 160 | 1/2 cup ice cream | 250 |
| 1/8 cup choc. covered raisins | 93 | 1/4 cup ranch dip with 1 cup fresh veggies | 170 | 1 piece apple pie (1/8th pie) | 296 |
| 5 medium shrimp with 1/4 cup cocktail sauce | 140 | 1/4 cup cheese fondue with 4-5 bread chunks or crackers | 200 | 1 cup pudding | 300 |

# MOVIE SNACKS
## Theater snacks are high in calories, fat, and sugar... be sensible, share with friends, and choose wisely

| FOOD | KCAL | FOOD | KCAL |
|---|---|---|---|
| **Popcorn in coconut oil** | | **Candy** | |
| kids (5 cups) | 300 | 1 package Whoppers (3 oz.) | 360 |
| small (7 cups) | 400 | 1 package Reese's Peanut Butter cups (2½ oz.) | 370 |
| medium (11 cups) | 650 | 1 package Raisinets (3 oz.) | 420 |
| medium (16 cups) | 900 | 1 package Buncha Crunch (3 oz.) | 480 |
| large (20 cups) | 1160 | 1 package Milk Duds (4 oz) | 490 |
| | | 1 Kit Kat (3½ oz.) | 500 |
| **Coconut oil w/ butter topping** | | 1 package Butterfinger Mini Bars (4 oz.) | 510 |
| | | 1 package Goobers (3½ oz.) | 530 |
| kids (5 cups) | 470 | 1 package Twizzlers strawberry (6oz) | 560 |
| small (7 cups) | 630 | 1 package Junior Mints (5½ oz.) | 620 |
| medium (11 cups) | 910 | 1 package Skittles (7 oz.) | 770 |
| medium (16 cups) | 1220 | 1 package plain M&M's (5½ oz.) | 770 |
| large (20 cups) | 1640 | 1 package Starburst Fruit Chews (7oz) | 800 |
| | | 1 package Reese's Pieces (8 oz.) | 1140 |
| **In vegetable shortening** | | | |
| small (7 cups) | 360 | **Soda** | |
| medium (11 cups) | 630 | 1 small diet soda (20 oz.) | 0 |
| large (20 cups) | 850 | 1 small soda (20 oz.) | 220 |

*Popcorn in a movie theater can be deceiving. Why? They use coconut oil which is twice as saturated as lard! The vegetable shortening, although not as healthy as "air popped" popcorn, is a better choice... however, only a few theaters offer vegetable shortening as an option. Source: M. F. Jacobson and J. G. Hurley,* Restaurant Confidential *(New York: Workman Publishing, 2002).*

| CANDY | | | | | |
|---|---|---|---|---|---|
| **CHOOSE OFTEN** | | **CHOOSE CAUTIOUSLY** | | **USE SPARINGLY** | |
| FOOD | KCAL | FOOD | KCAL | FOOD | KCAL |
| 2 Tootsie rolls | 55 | 10 peanut M & M's (or 20 plain) | 100 | 1 candy bar: Mars, Caramello, Heath, Whatchamacallit, Ghirardelli Milk Chocolate, Kit Kat, Nestle Crunch, Almond Joy | 250 |
| 1 handful (1/5 package) Skittles | 55 | 4 Hershey's Kisses | 105 | | |
| 3 Werther's Original | 60 | 17 jelly beans | 110 | 9 Hershey Hugs with Almonds | 230 |
| 3 Jolly Ranchers | 75 | 1 package Lifesavers | 110 | 4 assorted chocolates | 255 |
| 2 pieces Twizzlers licorice | 90 | 6 Starburst fruit chews | 120 | 1 candy bar: 5th Avenue, Twix, Snickers, NutRageous, Butterfinger, Reese's Peanut Butter Cups, 3 Musketeers, Baby Ruth | 300 |
| 9 Mento's | 90 | Junior Mints (1 small box) | 160 | | |
| | | York Peppermint Patty | 170 | | |
| | | 1 Milky Way Lite bar | 170 | | |

*Source: The nutrition information for all charts in the Flexible Meal Planner was taken from the USDA Nutrient Database for Standard Reference, Release 17. The nutrition information for specific restaurants or brands was taken from official restaurant websites and food labels based on research conducted through 2004. Nutrient values are subject to change. Some values have been averaged and/or estimated based on similar foods.*

# Strength Training

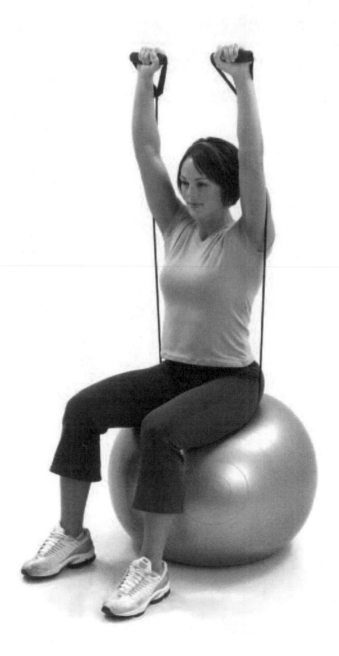

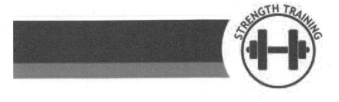

# INTRODUCTION

We custom-designed a progressive Core Strength Conditioning Program for you—and we put all eight weeks of it into an easy to follow flipchart. Each exercise comes complete with photos and a brief how-to description. Check your Daily Success Plan to find out which workout you should use each day.

For added resistance, loop the cord around your hand.

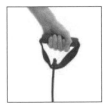 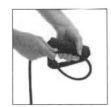 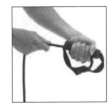

Core strength conditioning refers to strengthening the center, or "core," of your body. The core is comprised of over 35 muscles attached to the spine and pelvis, supporting and strengthening the rest of your body. As you strengthen and condition your core through this program, you'll improve balance, stability and posture, and you'll find that your whole body becomes more powerful and more resistant to injury. You'll be able to do more, and feel better, than you ever have before.

Now you have all the tools you need. . . so let's get started!

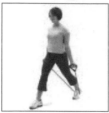 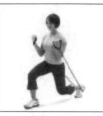

**2 sets of 15 reps each leg**

### Stationary Lunge with Bicep Curl
Stand with one leg forward about 4 feet, back straight, back foot on center of resistance cord; hold one handle in each hand, palms forward. Lower until front knee is bent to 90 degrees; kneecap shouldn't extend beyond toes. Exhale as you bend elbows and raise hands toward shoulder. Inhale as you raise legs and hands lower back down. Alternate one set on each leg.

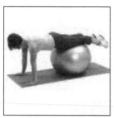 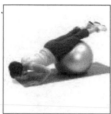

**2 sets of 15 reps**

### Push-up with Thighs on Ball
Kneel with ball in front of you; roll forward, walking on hands, until ball is under thighs; keep feet together; keep hands slightly wider than shoulder width apart. Lower slowly until face is 1-3 inches from floor; keep lower back straight; keep abs tight. Inhale as you lower your body, exhale as you lift.

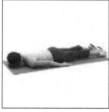 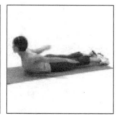

**2 sets of 15 reps**

### Prone Cobra
Lay face down on floor, arms at sides, palms down; contract lower back and lift chest about 6 inches; as you lift, turn palms so that your thumbs are facing the ceiling; keep head and neck in alignment. Keep shoelaces touching floor and gluteal muscles contracted throughout exercise; inhale as you raise your body, exhale as you lower it.

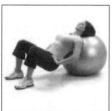 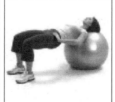

**2 sets of 15 reps**

### Bridge on Ball
Sit on ball; roll forward to rest upper back, neck and head on ball; bend knees to 90 degrees, feet on the floor hip width apart. Lift hips toward ceiling until parallel with floor, body in a straight line from head to knees. Inhale as you let hips sink down just above floor, then raise back up to starting position; as you raise hips, exhale and contract gluteal muscles.

# Level 1

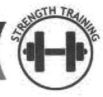

STRENGTH TRAINING

## WEEK 1

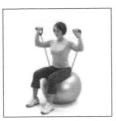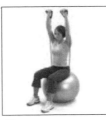

2 sets of 15 reps

### Seated Shoulder Press

Drape resistance cord over ball, handles even on each side; sit on center of resistance cord, back straight, abs tight, knees bent 90 degrees, feet hip width apart. Grasp one handle in each hand; raise arms to shoulder level, bent to 90 degrees, palms forward. Exhale as you raise arms until they come together over head. Inhale as you lower arms to shoulder level.

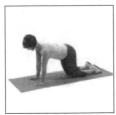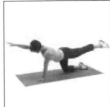

2 sets

### Spinal Balance

Start on hands and knees, face down; keep spine in neutral alignment, abs tight, lower back straight, shoulders down and back. Raise right leg straight out behind you, parallel with floor; raise left arm straight out ahead of you, also parallel with floor; hold for 10 seconds, then lower and change sides. Breathe deeply, keeping hips as level as possible.

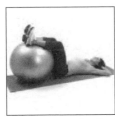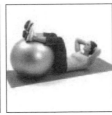

2 sets of 20 reps

### Crunch with Legs on Ball

Lay on floor, face up, ball underneath legs; keep legs relaxed on ball; press lower back toward floor and flex ab muscles; rest hands by ears, elbows far apart. Exhale as you curl up, lifting shoulder blades off floor; keep head and neck in neutral alignment, chin up off chest. Inhale as you lower body; keep abs engaged.

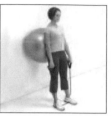 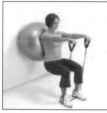

2 sets of 15 reps

## Wall Squat with Front Raise

Place ball against wall in curve of lower spine. Stand on resistance cord with both feet, one handle in each hand; keep feet shoulder width apart, abs tight, palms facing thighs. Bend knees and push hips back as if sitting in a chair, knees at 90 degrees; raise arms straight in front and exhale as you lower; keep knees behind shoelaces. Inhale and lower arms as you rise.

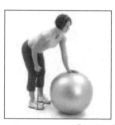 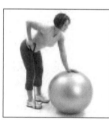

2 sets of 15 reps

## Chest Fly on Ball

Sit on ball; wrap resistance cord around upper back; walk feet forward until head, neck and upper shoulders are resting comfortably on ball. Cord should now be between upper back and ball. Lift hips; abs tight; one handle in each hand. Exhale as you bring handles straight up, palms facing each other; arms slightly bent at elbows. Inhale as you lower arms in line with shoulders.

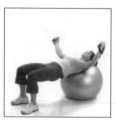 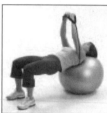

2 sets of 15 reps

## One-Arm Row on Ball

Place ball on floor. Step on resistance cord with both feet, outstep of right foot 6-8 inches from right handle. Bend from hips; place left hand on ball. Grab handle in right hand; keep abs tight, back straight, palm facing thigh. Exhale as you pull elbow up and back, close to body, neck in alignment, shoulders level. Inhale as you lower arm; alternate one set on each side.

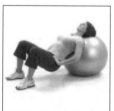 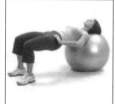

2 sets of 15 reps

## Bridge on Ball

Sit on ball; roll forward to rest upper back, neck and head on ball; bend knees to 90 degrees, feet on the floor hip width apart. Lift hips toward ceiling until parallel with floor, body in a straight line from head to knees. Inhale as you let hips sink down just above floor, then raise back up to starting position; as you raise hips, exhale and contract gluteal muscles.

# Level 1

STRENGTH TRAINING

## WEEK 2

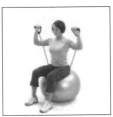 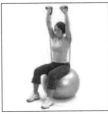

2 sets of 15 reps

### Seated Shoulder Press

Drape resistance cord over ball, handles even on each side; sit on center of resistance cord, back straight, abs tight, knees bent 90 degrees, feet hip width apart. Grasp one handle in each hand; raise arms to shoulder level, bent to 90 degrees, palms forward. Exhale as you raise arms until they come together over head. Inhale as you lower arms to shoulder level.

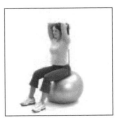 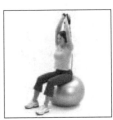

2 sets of 15 reps

### Seated Overhead Extension on Ball

Drape resistance cord over ball, handles even on each side; sit on center of cord, shoulders down, abs tight, one handle in each hand. Bring arms overhead, elbows close to ears, palms in. Inhale as you lower handles behind head to base of neck, elbows close to ears. Exhale as you extend arms back toward ceiling; focus on contracting tricep muscle.

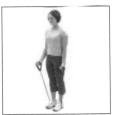 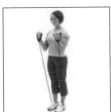

2 sets of 15 reps

### Standing Biceps Curl

Stand on center of resistance cord, feet hip width apart, toes forward; hold one handle in each hand, palms forward. Exhale and contract biceps, flexing elbows and bringing handles toward shoulders; inhale and lower handle back. Keep shoulders down and back throughout the exercise.

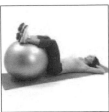 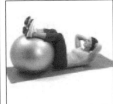

2 sets of 20 reps

### Crunch with Legs on Ball

Lay on floor, face up, ball underneath legs; keep legs relaxed on ball; press lower back toward floor and flex ab muscles; rest hands by ears, elbows far apart. Exhale as you curl up, lifting shoulder blades off floor; keep head and neck in neutral alignment, chin up off chest. Inhale as you lower body; keep abs engaged.

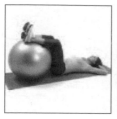 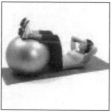

2 sets of 20 reps

### Crunch with Legs on Ball

Lay on floor, face up, ball underneath legs; keep legs relaxed on ball; press lower back toward floor and flex ab muscles; rest hands by ears, elbows far apart. Exhale as you curl up, lifting shoulder blades off floor; keep head and neck in neutral alignment, chin up off chest. Inhale as you lower body; keep abs engaged.

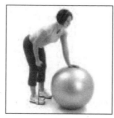 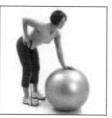

2 sets of 15 reps

### Bridge on Ball

Sit on ball; roll forward to rest upper back, neck and head on ball; bend knees to 90 degrees, feet on the floor hip width apart. Lift hips toward ceiling until parallel with floor, body in a straight line from head to knees. Inhale as you let hips sink down just above floor, then raise back up to starting position; as you raise hips, exhale and contract gluteal muscles.

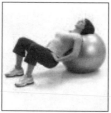 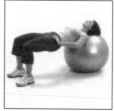

2 sets of 15 reps

### One-Arm Row on Ball

Place ball on floor. Step on resistance cord with both feet, outstep of right foot 6-8 inches from right handle. Bend from hips; place left hand on ball. Grab handle in right hand; keep abs tight, back straight, palm facing thigh. Exhale as you pull elbow up and back, close to body, neck in alignment, shoulders level. Inhale as you lower arm; alternate one set on each side.

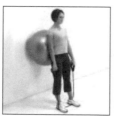 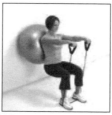

2 sets of 15 reps

### Wall Squat with Front Raise

Place ball against wall in curve of lower spine. Stand on resistance cord with both feet, one handle in each hand; keep feet shoulder width apart, abs tight, palms facing thighs. Bend knees and push hips back as if sitting in a chair; raise arms straight in front and exhale as you lower; keep knees behind shoelaces. Inhale and lower arms as you rise.

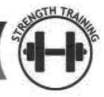

# Level 1

**STRENGTH TRAINING**

## WEEK 3

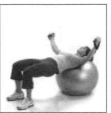 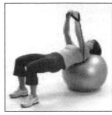

2 sets of 15 reps

### Chest Fly on Ball

Sit on ball; wrap resistance cord around upper back; walk feet forward until head, neck and upper shoulders are resting comfortably on ball. Cord should now be between upper back and ball. Lift hips; abs tight; one handle in each hand. Exhale as you bring handles straight up, palms facing each other; arms slightly bent at elbows. Inhale as you lower arms in line with shoulders.

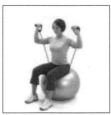 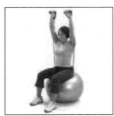

2 sets of 15 reps

### Seated Shoulder Press

Drape resistance cord over ball, handles even on each side; sit on center of resistance cord, back straight, abs tight, knees bent 90 degrees, feet hip width apart. Grasp one handle in each hand; raise arms to shoulder level, bent to 90 degrees, palms forward. Exhale as you raise arms until they come together over head. Inhale as you lower arms to shoulder level.

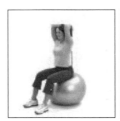 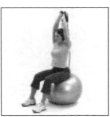

2 sets of 15 reps

### Seated Overhead Extension on Ball

Drape resistance cord over ball, handles even on each side; sit on center of cord, shoulders down, abs tight, one handle in each hand. Bring arms overhead, elbows close to ears, palms in. Inhale as you lower handles behind head to base of neck, elbows close to ears. Exhale as you extend arms back toward ceiling; focus on contracting tricep muscle.

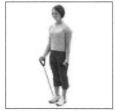 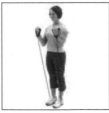

2 sets of 15 reps

### Standing Biceps Curl

Stand on center of resistance cord, feet hip width apart, toes forward; hold one handle in each hand, palms forward. Exhale and contract biceps, flexing elbows and bringing handles toward shoulders; inhale and lower handle back. Keep shoulders down and back throughout the exercise.

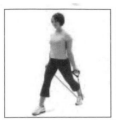 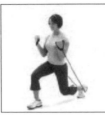

2 sets of 15 reps

### Stationary Lunge with Bicep Curl

Stand with one leg forward about 4 feet, back straight, back foot on center of resistance cord; hold one handle in each hand, palms forward. Lower until front knee is bent to 90 degrees; kneecap shouldn't extend beyond toes. Exhale as you bend elbows and raise hands toward shoulder. Inhale as you raise legs and hands lower back down. Alternate one set on each leg.

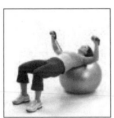 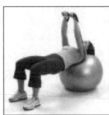

2 sets of 15 reps

### Chest Press on Ball

Sit on ball; wrap resistance cord around upper back; walk feet forward until head, neck and upper shoulders are resting comfortably on ball. Cord should now be between upper back and ball. Lift hips; abs tight; one handle in each hand. Bring arms up, elbows bent 90 degrees, palms facing toes; exhale as you raise handles over chest in an upside down V. Inhale as you lower handles back to 90 degrees.

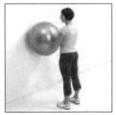 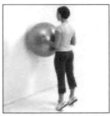

2 sets of 20 reps

### Standing Calf Raise with Ball Against Wall

Pick up ball and place it against wall, one hand on each side; feet together. Lean at an angle toward wall, pressing the ball between your chest and the wall. Exhale as you lift both heels upward slowly until you are balancing on your toes. Inhale as you lower slowly until heels touch floor; keep abs tight.

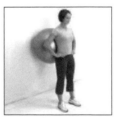 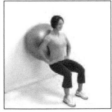

2 sets

### Isometric Wall Squat with Ball

Place ball against wall in curve of lower spine. Bend knees and push hips back as if sitting in a chair, knees at 90 degrees; hold contraction for 30 seconds; keep abs pulled inward toward the spine, knees and toes in alignment pointing forward. Remember to breath deeply as you hold, in through the nose and out through the mouth.

# Level 1

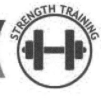

**STRENGTH TRAINING**

# WEEK 4

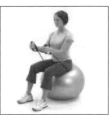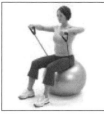

2 sets of 15 reps

## Seated Bent Arm Lateral Raise

Drape resistance cord over ball, handles even on each side; sit on center of resistance cord, back straight, abs tight, knees soft and toes forward. Grasp one handle in each hand, palms down; exhale as you lift arms to shoulder level, arms bent to 90 degrees. Inhale as you lower arms to starting position.

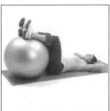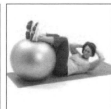

2 sets

## Spinal Balance

Start on hands and knees, face down; keep spine in neutral alignment, abs tight, lower back straight, shoulders down and back. Raise right leg straight out behind you, parallel with floor; raise left arm straight out ahead of you, also parallel with floor; hold for 10 seconds, then lower and change sides. Breathe deeply, keeping hips as level as possible.

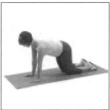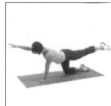

2 sets of 20 reps

## Oblique Crunch Legs on Ball

Lay on floor, face up, ball underneath legs, legs relaxed on ball; press lower back toward floor and flex ab muscles. Exhale as you curl upward, taking left shoulder blade off floor toward right knee; keep head and neck in neutral alignment, chin up off chest. Inhale as you lower body, keeping abs engaged. Repeat on other side.

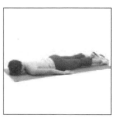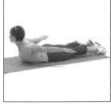

2 sets of 15 reps

## Prone Cobra

Lay face down on floor, arms at sides, palms down; contract lower back and lift chest about 6 inches; as you lift, turn palms so that your thumbs are facing the ceiling; keep head and neck in alignment. Keep shoelaces touching floor and gluteal muscles contracted throughout exercise; inhale as you raise your body, exhale as you lower it.

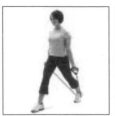 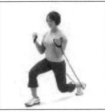

2 sets of 15 reps

### Stationary Lunge with Bicep Curl

Stand with one leg forward about 4 feet, back straight, back foot on center of resistance cord; hold one handle in each hand, palms forward. Lower until front knee is bent to 90 degrees; kneecap shouldn't extend beyond toes. Exhale as you bend elbows and raise hands toward shoulder. Inhale as you raise legs and hands lower back down. Alternate one set on each leg.

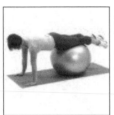 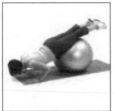

2 sets of 15 reps

### Push-up with Thighs on Ball

Kneel with ball in front of you; roll forward, walking on hands, until ball is under thighs; keep feet together; keep hands slightly wider than shoulder width apart. Lower slowly until face is 1-3 inches from floor; keep lower back straight; keep abs tight. Inhale as you lower your body, exhale as you lift.

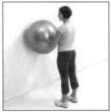 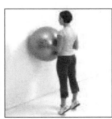

2 sets of 20 reps

### Standing Calf Raise with Ball Against Wall

Pick up ball and place it against wall, one hand on each side; feet together. Lean at an angle toward wall, pressing the ball between your chest and the wall. Exhale as you lift both heels upward slowly until you are balancing on your toes. Inhale as you lower slowly until heels touch floor; keep abs tight.

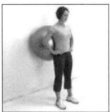 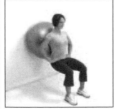

2 sets

### Isometric Wall Squat with Ball

Place ball against wall in curve of lower spine. Bend knees and push hips back as if sitting in a chair, knees at 90 degrees; hold contraction for 30 seconds; keep abs pulled inward toward the spine, knees and toes in alignment pointing forward. Remember to breath deeply as you hold, in through the nose and out through the mouth.

# Level 1 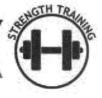 **WEEK 5**

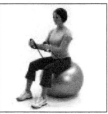 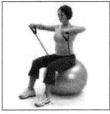

2 sets of 15 reps

### Seated Bent Arm Lateral Raise

Drape resistance cord over ball, handles even on each side; sit on center of resistance cord, back straight, abs tight, knees soft and toes forward. Grasp one handle in each hand, palms down; exhale as you lift arms to shoulder level, arms bent to 90 degrees. Inhale as you lower arms to starting position.

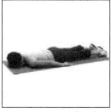 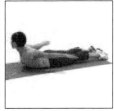

2 sets of 15 reps

### Prone Cobra

Lay face down on floor, arms at sides, palms down; contract lower back and lift chest about 6 inches; as you lift, turn palms so that your thumbs are facing the ceiling; keep head and neck in alignment. Keep shoelaces touching floor and gluteal muscles contracted throughout exercise; inhale as you raise your body, exhale as you lower it.

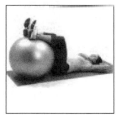 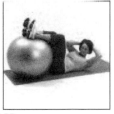

2 sets of 20 reps

### Oblique Crunch Legs on Ball

Lay on floor, face up, ball underneath legs, legs relaxed on ball; press lower back toward floor and flex ab muscles. Exhale as you curl upward, taking left shoulder blade off floor toward right knee; keep head and neck in neutral alignment, chin up off chest. Inhale as you lower body, keeping abs engaged. Repeat on other side.

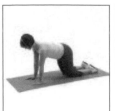
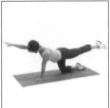

2 sets

### Spinal Balance

Start on hands and knees, face down; keep spine in neutral alignment, abs tight, lower back straight, shoulders down and back. Raise right leg straight out behind you, parallel with floor; raise left arm straight out ahead of you, also parallel with floor; hold for 10 seconds, then lower and change sides. Breathe deeply, keeping hips as level as possible.

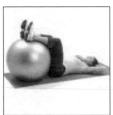
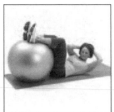

2 sets of 20 reps

### Oblique Crunch Legs on Ball

Lay on floor, face up, ball underneath legs, legs relaxed on ball; press lower back toward floor and flex ab muscles. Exhale as you curl upward, taking left shoulder blade off floor toward right knee; keep head and neck in neutral alignment, chin up off chest. Inhale as you lower body, keeping abs engaged. Repeat on other side.

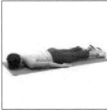
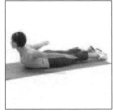

2 sets of 15 reps

### Prone Cobra

Lay face down on floor, arms at sides, palms down; contract lower back and lift chest about 6 inches; as you lift, turn palms so that your thumbs are facing the ceiling; keep head and neck in alignment. Keep shoelaces touching floor and gluteal muscles contracted throughout exercise; inhale as you raise your body, exhale as you lower it.

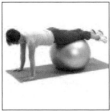
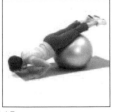

2 sets of 15 reps

### Push-up with Thighs on Ball

Kneel with ball in front of you; roll forward, walking on hands, until ball is under thighs; keep feet together; keep hands slightly wider than shoulder width apart. Lower slowly until face is 1-3 inches from floor; keep lower back straight; keep abs tight. Inhale as you lower your body, exhale as you lift.

# Level 1

STRENGTH TRAINING

## WEEK 6

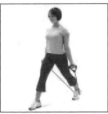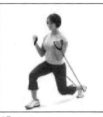

2 sets of 15 reps

### Stationary Lunge with Bicep Curl

Stand with one leg forward about 4 feet, back straight, back foot on center of resistance cord; hold one handle in each hand, palms forward. Lower until front knee is bent to 90 degrees; kneecap shouldn't extend beyond toes. Exhale as you bend elbows and raise hands toward shoulder. Inhale as you raise legs and hands lower back down. Alternate one set on each leg.

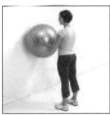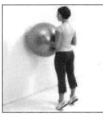

2 sets of 20 reps

### Standing Calf Raise with Ball Against Wall

Pick up ball and place it against wall, one hand on each side; feet together. Lean at an angle toward wall, pressing the ball between your chest and the wall. Exhale as you lift both heels upward slowly until you are balancing on your toes. Inhale as you lower slowly until heels touch floor; keep abs tight.

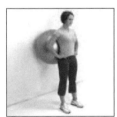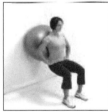

2 sets

### Isometric Wall Squat with Ball

Place ball against wall in curve of lower spine. Bend knees and push hips back as if sitting in a chair, knees at 90 degrees; hold contraction for 30 seconds; keep abs pulled inward toward the spine, knees and toes in alignment pointing forward. Remember to breath deeply as you hold, in through the nose and out through the mouth.

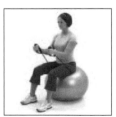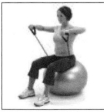

2 sets of 15 reps

### Seated Bent Arm Lateral Raise

Drape resistance cord over ball, handles even on each side; sit on center of resistance cord, back straight, abs tight, knees soft and toes forward. Grasp one handle in each hand, palms down; exhale as you lift arms to shoulder level, arms bent to 90 degrees. Inhale as you lower arms to starting position.

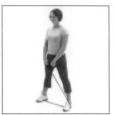 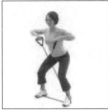

2 sets of 15 reps

## Wide Squat with Upright Row

Stand on resistance cord with feet wider than shoulder width; grab right handle with left hand and left handle with right hand: when you raise the cord it should form an X. Keep knees and toes turned out 45 degrees, palms facing thighs, knees bent. Exhale as you bend legs and lower body; bring hands to shoulder level; keep hands close together, shoulders down; slightly squeeze the blades. Inhale as you stand up; lower arms to starting position.

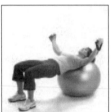 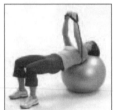

2 sets of 15 reps

## Chest Fly on Ball

Sit on ball; wrap resistance cord around upper back; walk feet forward until head, neck and upper shoulders are resting comfortably on ball. Cord should now be between upper back and ball. Lift hips; abs tight; one handle in each hand. Exhale as you bring handles straight up, palms facing each other; arms slightly bent at elbows. Inhale as you lower arms in line with shoulders.

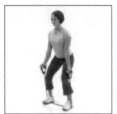 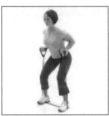

2 sets of 15 reps

## Bent Over Row

Stand on center of resistance cord with feet hip width apart; knees and toes in alignment facing forward; one handle in each hand with palms facing forward. Bend hips to 45 degree angle; extend the arms straight out in front of you towards the floor. Using your back muscles, exhale and pull the handles toward your ribs, inhale and lower back down.

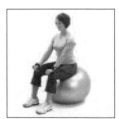 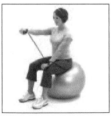

2 sets of 15 reps

## Alternating Front Raise

Drape resistance cord over ball, handles even on each side; sit on center of resistance cord, back straight, abs tight, knees bent 90 degrees, feet hip width apart. Grasp one handle in each hand, hands on knees, palms down. Exhale as you lift one arm forward to shoulder height; don't lock elbow. Inhale as you lower slowly. Repeat with opposite arm.

# Level 1

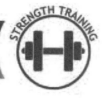
STRENGTH TRAINING

## WEEK 7

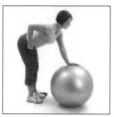 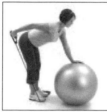

**2 sets of 15 reps**

### Arm Tricep Kickback on Ball

Stand on center of resistance cord, feet hip width apart, ball in front of you; hold one handle in right hand. Bend from hips, left hand on ball, abs tight, knees soft. Pull right elbow up to rib cage, in line with shoulder, palm in. Exhale as you straighten arm from elbow joint until arm is parallel to floor. Inhale as you bring hand back toward floor, elbow in place. Alternate one set on each side.

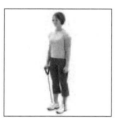 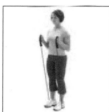

**2 sets of 15 reps**

### Standing Hammer Curls

Stand on center of resistance cord, feet hip width apart, toes forward; hold one handle in each hand, palms in. Exhale and contract biceps, flexing elbows and bringing handles toward shoulders; inhale and lower handle back. Keep shoulders down and back throughout the exercise.

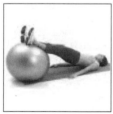 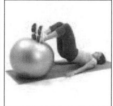

**2 sets of 15 reps**

### Hamstring Curl on Ball

Lie on floor, face up, ball directly under calves and heels, hands at sides with palms down. Contract gluteal muscles; lift hips about 3 inches off floor; keep spine in neutral alignment and abs tight; press heels deep into ball as you roll in and out. When legs are extended, keep knees soft. Exhale as you contract hamstrings, pulling ball in toward gluteal muscles; inhale as you roll back to starting position.

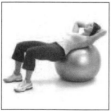 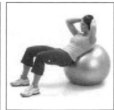

**2 sets of 20 reps**

### Basic Trunk Lift

Sit on ball; walk feet forward until ball is in curve of spine, feet hip width apart, abs tight; rest hands by ears, elbows far apart. Exhale as you curl up, lifting shoulder blades off ball; keep head and neck in neutral alignment, chin up off chest. Inhale as you lower your body; keep abs engaged.

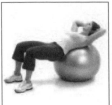 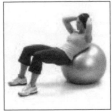

2 sets of 20 reps

### Basic Trunk Lift

Sit on ball; walk feet forward until ball is in curve of spine, feet hip width apart, abs tight; rest hands by ears, elbows far apart. Exhale as you curl up, lifting shoulder blades off ball; keep head and neck in neutral alignment, chin up off chest. Inhale as you lower your body; keep abs engaged.

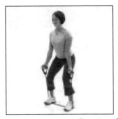 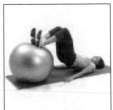

2 sets of 15 reps

### Hamstring Curl on Ball

Lie on floor, face up, ball directly under calves and heels, hands at sides with palms down. Contract gluteal muscles; lift hips about 3 inches off floor; keep spine in neutral alignment and abs tight; press heels deep into ball as you roll in and out. When legs are extended, keep knees soft. Exhale as you contract hamstrings, pulling ball in toward gluteal muscles; inhale as you roll back to starting position.

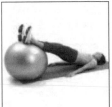 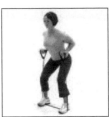

2 sets of 15 reps

### Bent Over Row

Stand on center of resistance cord with feet hip width apart; knees and toes in alignment facing forward; one handle in each hand with palms facing forward. Bend hips to 45 degree angle; extend the arms straight out in front of you towards the floor. Using your back muscles, exhale and pull the handles toward your ribs, inhale and lower back down.

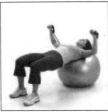 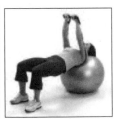

2 sets of 15 reps

### Chest Press on Ball

Sit on ball; wrap resistance cord around upper back; walk feet forward until head, neck and upper shoulders are resting comfortably on ball. Cord should now be between upper back and ball. Lift hips; abs tight; one handle in each hand. Bring arms up, elbows bent 90 degrees, palms facing toes; exhale as you raise handles over chest in an upside down V. Inhale as you lower handles back to 90 degrees.

# Level 1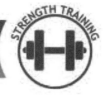

## WEEK 8

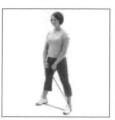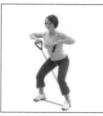

2 sets of 15 reps

### Wide Squat with Upright Row

Stand on resistance cord with feet wider than shoulder width; grab right handle with left hand and left handle with right hand: when you raise the cord it should form an X. Keep knees and toes turned out 45 degrees, palms facing thighs, knees bent. Exhale as you bend legs and lower body; bring hands to shoulder level; keep hands close together, shoulders down; slightly squeeze the blades. Inhale as you stand up; lower arms to starting position.

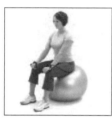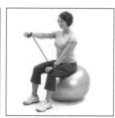

2 sets of 15 reps

### Alternating Front Raise

Drape resistance cord over ball, handles even on each side; sit on center of resistance cord, back straight, abs tight, knees bent 90 degrees, feet hip width apart. Grasp one handle in each hand, hands on knees, palms down. Exhale as you lift one arm forward to shoulder height; don't lock elbow. Inhale as you lower slowly. Repeat with opposite arm.

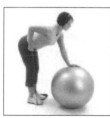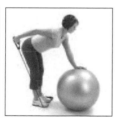

2 sets of 15 reps

### Arm Tricep Kickback on Ball

Stand on center of resistance cord, feet hip width apart, ball in front of you; hold one handle in right hand. Bend from hips, left hand on ball, abs tight, knees soft. Pull right elbow up to rib cage, in line with shoulder, palm in. Exhale as you straighten arm from elbow joint until arm is parallel to floor. Inhale as you bring hand back toward floor, elbow in place. Alternate one set on each side.

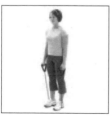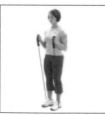

2 sets of 15 reps

### Standing Hammer Curls

Stand on center of resistance cord, feet hip width apart, toes forward; hold one handle in each hand, palms in. Exhale and contract biceps, flexing elbows and bringing handles toward shoulders; inhale and lower handle back. Keep shoulders down and back throughout the exercise.

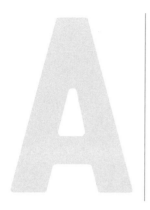

# Appendix

**KEY POINTS:**

Recipes | Tips for Eating Away from Home | Questions and Answers | Testimonials

## Recipes

### Steamed Salmon with Black Bean Sauce (Option 1)

240 calories per 4-ounce serving

**Sauce**

| | |
|---|---|
| ⅓ cup | **fermented black beans** |
| 2 Tbs. | **soy sauce** |
| 2 tsp. | **sugar** |
| 1 tsp. | **sesame oil** |
| 2 Tbs. | **rice vinegar** |
| 1 rounded Tbs. | **cornstarch** |
| ⅓ cup | **water** |

**Salmon**

| | |
|---|---|
| 2 pounds | **salmon fillets** |
| 4 | **scallions, chopped in 1-inch pieces** |

1. Combine sauce ingredients together in small saucepan. Heat to boiling, stirring constantly until thickened. Set aside.
2. Spray baking sheet with nonstick cooking spray and lay salmon steaks on sheet. Top with scallions. Broil on high 7–10 minutes or until fish flakes easily with fork.
3. Drizzle salmon with black bean sauce and serve. Serves 4.

## Creole Pork Tenderloin (Option 2)

231 calories per 4-ounce serving

approximately

| | |
|---|---|
| 2 lbs. | Lean pork tenderloin |
| 1 tsp. | garlic salt or garlic powder |
| 1 tsp. | onion powder |
| 1 tsp. | cayenne |
| | Fresh ground pepper |
| 1–2 tsp. | olive oil |

1. Rub tenderloin with all seasonings.
2. Add small amount of oil in large skillet, sear tenderloin over medium-high heat on all sides. Place in baking dish and bake at 350 degree oven for approximately 30 minutes. Check for internal temperature of 170 degrees. Serves 4 (4 oz.) servings.

## Apple Jicama Salsa

| | |
|---|---|
| 2 | Granny Smith apples, cored and diced |
| 1 | jicama, peeled and diced (Jicama looks like a large, round potato with a brown peel. Cut jicama in half and then into quarters, giving you smaller pieces to peel. Use a paring knife or vegetable peeler and remove the thick, brown peel. The jicama has a slightly sweet flavor—a cross between an apple and a potato.) |
| ½ | red onion, minced |
| 3 Tbs. | chopped fresh cilantro |
| 2 Tbs. | lime juice |
| 1 tsp. | salt |
| | Fresh ground pepper to taste |
| ½ tsp. | red pepper |

1. Combine all ingredients and stir thoroughly. Makes approximately 4 cups. Serve alongside Creole Pork Tenderloin.

## Chicken Enchiladas (Option 3)

290 calories per enchilada

| | |
|---|---|
| 4 | boneless, skinless chicken breasts |
| 1 Tbs. | olive oil |
| ½ tsp | cumin |
| 2 tsp. | minced garlic cloves |
| 1 | onion, chopped |
| 1 | jalapeno, seeded and minced |
| | Salt and pepper to taste |
| 1 (14 oz.) can | fat-free refried beans |
| 8 | whole-wheat tortillas |
| 1 (10 oz.) can | enchilada sauce |
| 4 oz. | shredded low-fat cheddar cheese |
| ½ cup | fat-free sour cream |

1. Boil chicken breasts in water until done. Remove, let cool, and shred or thinly slice. Heat oil in skillet. Add cumin, garlic, onion, and jalapeno. Stir fry 3 minutes. Add cooked chicken, salt and pepper, and red pepper. Simmer to warm through.
2. Fill tortillas with equal portions of refried beans and chicken. Roll up and place in a baking dish large enough to fit all 8 enchiladas. Pour enchilada sauce over the top and sprinkle with shredded cheese. Bake at 350 degrees for approximately 20 minutes or until cheese is melted and enchiladas are warmed through. Serve each with a dollop of sour cream and your favorite salsa. A homemade salsa recipe follows. Makes 8 enchiladas.

## Salsa

| | |
|---|---|
| 6 | **tomatoes** |
| ½ | **red onion, minced** |
| ½ bunch | **fresh cilantro** |
| 1 | **jalapeno, seeds removed and minced** |
| | **juice of 3 limes** |
| | **salt and pepper to taste** |

1. Combine all ingredients and serve. Makes about 6 cups.

## Roasted Tomato Pasta (Option 5)

335 calories per 1-cup serving

| | |
|---|---|
| 1 lb. | **pasta of choice** |
| 12 | **Roma tomatoes or carton of cherry or grape tomatoes** |
| ⅓ cup | **olive oil** |
| ½ cup | **minced fresh basil or 1 Tbs. dried** |
| ¼ cup | **minced fresh oregano or 1 tsp. dried** |
| 2 Tbs. | **minced thyme or 2 tsp. dried** |
| 1–2 tsp. | **salt** |
| 1 tsp. | **pepper** |
| 1 tsp. | **minced garlic** |
| 1 tsp. | **red pepper flakes** |
| ¼ cup | **grated Parmesan cheese** |

1. Prepare pasta according to package directions. Set aside. Meanwhile prepare tomatoes.
2. Cut Roma tomatoes in half and place on large baking sheet. If you're using cherry tomatoes or grape tomatoes, there is no need to cut them in half. Place remaining ingredients except Parmesan on baking pan and stir toma-

toes around to mix herbs and seasonings.
3. Broil for 5–7 minutes or until tomatoes are softened and slightly roasted. Pour entire mixture over pasta. Use a rubber scraper to get every bit of the seasoning from the baking sheet. Sprinkle with Parmesan cheese and serve. Makes approximately 8 cups.

## Chicken Divan (Option 16)

350 calories per 1½ cupserving

| | |
|---|---|
| 1½ lbs. | **boneless, skinless chicken breasts, diced** |
| 1 (10 oz.) package | **frozen broccoli spears, rinsed and drained** |
| 1 can | **reduced-fat cream of mushroom soup** |
| 2 Tbs. | **Parmesan cheese** |

Place diced chicken breasts in baking dish. Lay broccoli spears over chicken. Spread mushroom soup over top. Bake at 350 degrees for 30 minutes or until chicken is cooked through. Sprinkle with Parmesan cheese and brown in oven, if desired. Serves 4.

## Fish with Orange-Rosemary Sauce (Option 17)

198 calories per 4-ounce serving

| | |
|---|---|
| 4 (8 oz.) | **fish fillets** |

### Sauce

| | |
|---|---|
| 1 cup | orange-juice concentrate |
| ½ cup | water |
| 4 | shallots, minced, or 1/2 red onion, minced |
| 2 Tbs. | lemon juice |
| 2 Tbs. | fresh rosemary sprigs or 1–2 tsp. dried |
| | Salt and pepper to taste |

1. Prepare fillets as desired: steam, pan fry, broil, or grill until flesh flakes easily with a fork.
2. Meanwhile prepare sauce. Combine all ingredients in saucepan. Bring to a boil. Lower heat, simmer, and let reduce by a third. Pour over cooked fish. Serves 4.

## Steak Fajitas (Option 19)

315 calories per fajita

### Fajita Marinade

| | |
|---|---|
| 4 tsp. | minced garlic |
| ⅓ cup | lime juice |
| 2 Tbs. | soy sauce |
| ⅓ cup | red wine vinegar |
| 1 | jalapeno, cut in half |
| ½ tsp. | each salt and pepper |
| 1 ½ lb. | skirt or sirloin steaks, cut very thin across the grain |
| 1 Tbs. | olive oil |
| 1 | each red, green, and yellow bell pepper, cut into strips |
| 1 | onion, cut into strips |
| 8 oz. | mushrooms, sliced (optional) |
| 8 | whole-wheat tortillas |
| 2 cups | shredded low-fat cheddar cheese |
| 2 | tomatoes, diced |
| 2 cups | shredded lettuce |
| | Guacamole (recipe follows) |
| | Salsa (recipe follows) |

1. Combine marinade ingredients together in a large zip-lock–style bag. Add meat and let marinate overnight if possible. Remove meat from marinade and pat meat dry with paper towels. Discard marinade.
2. Heat oil in large skillet over high heat. Cook peppers and onions first. Stir fry on high heat to keep pan dry and vegetables browning. Remove when vegetables are lightly browned. Then remove vegetables to a platter and set aside.
3. Cook mushrooms in the same manner. Remove to platter with vegetables. Add additional oil if needed while cooking. Add meat and continue to stir fry on high heat just until meat is done.
4. Return vegetables to pan and stir to warm through. Season with salt and pepper and take the pan to the table. Let everyone assemble their fajitas. Have tortillas, cheese, diced tomatoes, lettuce, guacamole, and salsa in different dishes at the table. Enjoy! By the way, chicken can be substituted for the steak; follow the same directions but stir fry until the chicken is completely cooked through. Makes 8 fajitas.

## Guacamole

| 3 | ripe avocados |
| 2 oz. | fat-free cream cheese |
| | Salt and pepper to taste |

1. Mix all ingredients together until smooth. Makes approximately 1 cup.

## Salsa

| 3 | tomatoes |
| $^1/_4$ | red onion, minced |
| $^1/_4$ bunch | fresh cilantro |
| $^1/_2$ | jalapeno, seeds removed and minced |
| $^1/_4$ cup | lime juice |
| | salt and pepper to taste |

1. Combine all ingredients and serve. Makes about 3 cups.

## Spicy Black Beans

| 1 Tbs. | olive oil |
| 1 medium | onion, chopped |
| 2 cloves | garlic, minced |
| 2 tsp. | chili powder |
| 1 tsp. | cumin |
| 1 tsp. | crushed red pepper |
| 2 (15 oz.) cans | black beans, rinsed or drained |
| $^1/_4$ cup | loosely packed chopped cilantro |
| | Salt and pepper to taste |
| | Lime wedges |

1. Heat oil in skillet; add garlic and onion. Stir fry until onion softens, about 5 minutes. Stir in chili powder, cumin, and crushed red pepper; cook 30 seconds. Stir in beans and reduce heat to low. Simmer, uncovered, 10 minutes.

2. Sprinkle with cilantro and season with salt and pepper. Serve with lime wedges. Makes about 4 cups.

## Mediterranean Pesto Chicken (Option 20)

270 calories per 1-breast serving

| | |
|---|---|
| 1 Tbs. | **olive oil** |
| 1 tsp. | **minced garlic** |
| 1 ½ lbs. | **boneless, skinless chicken breasts** |
| | **Salt and pepper** |
| 1 Tbs. | **capers (optional)** |
| ¼ cup | **Parmesan cheese** |

### Pesto Sauce

| | |
|---|---|
| 2 Tbs. | **olive oil** |
| 1 cup | **fresh basil leaves** |
| ½ tsp. | **minced garlic** |
| 1 Tbs. | **pine nuts or almonds** |

1. Heat olive oil in large skillet. Add garlic and chicken. Sauté over medium heat to lightly brown chicken. Season with salt and pepper and capers. Cover and reduce heat to medium low. Simmer until chicken is cooked through; turn chicken occasionally.
2. Meanwhile, prepare Pesto Sauce. Place all Pesto Sauce ingredients in a food processor and combine until smooth. (Bottled Pesto Sauce may be purchased at the grocery store, usually in the produce department.) Add to chicken and stir to coat chicken breasts.
3. Transfer to serving dish, sprinkle with Parmesan cheese, and serve. Serves 4.

*These bonus Losing It! recipes are not only delicious, but healthy alternatives for if and when you get bored with the 21 dinner options on the Flexible Meal Planner. To incorporate these recipes into the meal plan, simply note the calories per serving, how many servings you plan to eat (think small), and how many calories you are allowed for that specific meal. If that sounds too complicated, simply use these recipes for fun! It is always great to try something new with your family and friends. And these recipes offer a valuable added bonus . . . they're healthy!*

## Spaghetti with Sauce

300 calories per 1-cup serving

| | |
|---|---|
| 1 Tbsp. | **olive oil** |
| 1–2 tsp. | **minced garlic** |
| 1 | **yellow, white or red onion, chopped** |
| 1 lb. | **lean ground beef** |
| 2 | **(15-oz.) can Italian-flavored, diced, stewed tomatoes, or crushed tomatoes** |
| 1 | **(6-oz.) can tomato paste** |
| 1 | **(29-oz.) can tomato sauce** |
| | **salt and pepper to taste** |
| 2 Tbsp. | **fresh, minced basil, or 1–2 tsp. dried** |
| 1 Tbsp. | **fresh, minced oregano, or 1 tsp. dried** |
| 2 Tbsp. | **balsamic vinegar, optional** |
| 1 lb. | **pasta of choice, cook following package directions** |
| ¼ cup | **Parmesan cheese** |

1. Heat olive oil in large skillet or saucepan. Add garlic and onion, sauté 1 minute. Add ground beef and cook until browned. Add remaining ingredients and let simmer 15–20 minutes. Prepare pasta.
2. When pasta is done, drain and toss with sauce. Sprinkle with cheese and serve.
   Makes approximately 5 cups.

## Pasta Primavera

225 calories per 1-cup serving

| | |
|---|---|
| 16 oz. | linguine |
| 1 Tbsp. | butter |
| 2–3 tsp. | minced garlic |
| 2 | green onions, chopped; white separated from green chive |
| 8 oz. | sliced mushrooms |
| 1 cup | chopped broccoli florets |
| 8 | asparagus spears, cut into 1" pieces |
| 2 | cups snow peas |
| 1 | red bell pepper, sliced julienne |
| 3 Tbsp. | chopped, fresh basil or 1 Tbsp. dried basil |
| | salt and pepper to taste |
| 3 cups | cooked, cubed chicken or 1 lb. cooked shrimp |
| 1/4 cup | half-and-half |
| 1/2 cup | freshly grated Parmesan cheese |

1. Cook linguine according to package directions.
2. Meanwhile, melt butter in a large skillet. Add garlic and white part of green onions; cook for 30 seconds. Add mushrooms and broccoli. Sauté 3 minutes or until mushrooms are softened. Add asparagus, snow peas, bell pepper, basil, and salt and pepper. Cook and stir until vegetables are slightly tender.
3. Toss vegetables and chicken or shrimp with linguine, add half-and-half. Sprinkle with Parmesan cheese. Let set a few minutes before serving. Makes 12 cups.

## Tender Turkey Breast with Herbs

270 calories per 1-cup serving

| | |
|---|---|
| 1/2 cup | olive oil |
| 1/4 cup | lemon juice |
| 2 Tbsp. | fresh basil, chopped or 1 Tbsp. dried |
| 1 Tbsp. | fresh oregano, chopped or 1 tsp. dried |
| 1 Tbsp. | fresh thyme, chopped or 1 tsp. dried |
| | salt and pepper to taste |
| 1 1/2 lb. | turkey breast, sliced in 1-in. strips |

1. In a gallon resealable bag, combine all ingredients. Shake to coat turkey with herbs. Let marinate in refrigerator at least an hour or overnight.
2. Pour 1 Tbsp. olive oil in large baking pan. Remove turkey from marinade and place on oiled pan. Discard marinade. Bake at 350° F for 10–15 minutes or until turkey is cooked through. Stir and turn turkey once halfway through cooking time. Serves 4 (5-oz. servings).

## Broiled or Grilled Lemon Chicken with Roasted Veggies

330 calories per 1½-cup cerving

**Marinade***

|  | lemon zest of one lemon |
| 1 cup | lemon juice |
| ½ cup | olive oil |
|  | salt and pepper to taste |
| 1 tsp. | minced garlic |

**Meat**

| 1½ lbs. | boneless, skinless chicken breasts |

**Vegetables**

| 1 bunch | broccoli, 1 crookneck or zucchini squash, all cut into large, bite-size chunks |
| 1 | russet or 2 red potatoes, sliced ¼" or thinner for equal cooking time |
| 8 oz. | whole mushrooms |

1. Mix marinade ingredients together in a large resealable bag. Add chicken and vegetables and let marinate 1 hour or as long as overnight, turning bag and moving vegetables around occasionally.
2. Remove chicken and vegetables from marinade and place on a cookie sheet sprayed with a non-stick spray. Discard marinade. Roast meat and vegetables in oven at 375° F for 20–30 minutes or until chicken is cooked through. Stir and turn occasionally. When meat is done, season to taste and serve. Serves 4.

*This marinade is also delicious with fish.

## Sliced, Seasoned Chicken over Spinach Salad

360 calories per 3-cup cerving

| 1 Tbsp. | olive oil |
| 1 tsp. | minced garlic |
| 1½ lbs. | boneless, skinless chicken breasts, sliced in 1"x3" strips |

**Dressing**

| ¼ cup | balsamic vinegar |
| ¼ cup | olive oil |
| 2 Tbsp. | Dijon mustard |
| 1 Tbsp. | each, minced basil and thyme or 1 tsp. each, dried |
| 1 tsp. | minced garlic |
|  | salt and pepper to taste |
| 1 lb. | fresh spinach salad greens, washed and rinsed well |
| 1 large | tomato, sliced |
| 4 | green onions, sliced |

1. Heat oil and garlic in skillet, sauté 30 seconds. Add chicken and stir-fry until lightly browned and cooked through, approximately 3–5 minutes.
2. When chicken is cooked through, transfer to a plate and cool. While chicken is cooling, whisk together dressing ingredients.
3. Discard coarse stems from spinach, toss with tomato and green onions. Arrange chicken over spinach salad and drizzle with dressing. Serves 4.

## Orange Chicken

265 calories per 1-cup serving

| | |
|---|---|
| ¹/₄ cup | **fat-free chicken broth** |
| 3 Tbsp. | **hoisin sauce** |
| 2 Tbsp. | **apricot preserves** |
| 2 tsp. | **soy sauce** |
| 1 tsp. | **orange zest** |
| 2 large | oranges |
| 3 Tbsp. | **chopped, fresh cilantro** |
| 1 Tbsp. | **olive oil** |
| 1¹/₂ lbs. | **boneless, skinless chicken breasts, cut into large chunks** |

1. In a small bowl, combine first five ingredients. Set aside.
2. Peel and coarsely chop oranges, remove seeds. In a large bowl, gently toss oranges with cilantro. Set aside.
3. Heat olive oil in skillet. Add chicken pieces and sauté 2–5 minutes or until lightly browned. Pour hoisin sauce mixture over chicken; simmer 5 minutes. Sauce will reduce while simmering and will create a glaze for chicken. Remove to platter, serve with orange cilantro mixture. Makes approximately 4½ cups.

## Soft Chicken Tacos with Black Beans

280 calories per taco

| | |
|---|---|
| 4 | **chicken breasts** |
| 1 Tbsp. | **olive oil** |
| ¹/₂ tsp. | **cumin** |
| 2 tsp. | **minced garlic cloves** |
| 1 | **onion, chopped** |
| 2 | **bell peppers, chopped** |
| 2 | **tomatoes, chopped** |
| 1 (14-oz.) can | **black beans, drained and rinsed** |
| | **juice of 1 lime** |
| | **salt and pepper to taste** |
| | **red pepper to taste** |
| 8 | **whole-wheat tortillas** |
| 4 oz. | **shredded low-fat cheddar cheese** |
| 2 | **tomatoes, chopped** |
| 2 cups | **shredded lettuce** |
| ¹/₂ cup | **low-fat sour cream** |

1. Boil chicken breasts in water approximately 20 minutes or until done. Remove, let cool and shred or thinly slice. (A whole chicken can be cooked and shredded as well). Heat oil in skillet. Add cumin, garlic, onion and bell peppers; stir-fry 3 minutes. Add cooked chicken, tomatoes, black beans, lime, salt and pepper, and red pepper. Simmer to warm through.
2. Fill tortillas with equal portions of chicken mixture; top each with ½ oz. cheddar cheese, tomatoes, lettuce, and 1 Tbsp. sour cream. Serve with salsa. Makes 8 tacos.

## Salsa

| | |
|---|---|
| 3 | tomatoes |
| ¹/₄ | red onion, minced |
| ¹/₄ bunch | fresh cilantro, use less if you like |
| ¹/₂ | jalapeno, seeds removed and minced |
| ¹/₄ cup | lime juice |
| | salt and pepper to taste |

1. Combine all ingredients and serve. Makes about 3 cups.

## Tiny Spicy Chicken

320 calories per 1-cup serving

| | |
|---|---|
| 1¹/₂ lbs. | boneless, skinless chicken breast, cut into bite-size pieces |
| 1 | egg white |
| 1¹/₂ Tbsp. | cornstarch |
| | dash salt |
| 2–4 Tbsp. | olive oil |
| 2 tsp. | minced garlic |
| 2 tsp. | minced ginger root |
| 2 tsp. | red pepper flakes |
| 3 | green onions, minced |
| ¹/₃–¹/₂ cup | catsup |
| 1 tsp. | hot chili oil |
| 2 Tbsp. | soy sauce |
| 2–3 Tbsp. | brown sugar |
| ¹/₄–¹/₂ tsp. | sesame oil (optional) |
| 1 Tbsp. | cornstarch |
| | garlic-salt and pepper to taste |

1. Marinate chicken in egg white, cornstarch and salt. Let set 10–15 minutes.
2. Heat 2 Tbsp. oil in skillet. Add garlic, ginger root, red pepper flakes and green onions. Stir-fry 1 minute. Add chicken and cook 4–5 minutes until cooked through. Remove chicken from skillet and set aside.
3. Reduce heat; add 1 Tbsp. olive oil, catsup and hot chili oil; stir until blended. In a separate bowl, mix soy sauce, sugar, sherry, sesame oil (if desired) and cornstarch.
4. Return chicken to skillet and pour sauce over; simmer and stir until sauce thickens. Makes approximately 5 cups.

## Kung Pao Chicken

350 calories per ¼-cup serving

| | |
|---|---|
| 1 Tbsp. | olive oil |
| 1 lb. | boneless, skinless chicken breasts, cut into bite-size pieces |
| 3 tsp. | minced garlic |
| 1 Tbsp. | minced ginger root |
| 1 bunch | green onion, chopped; separate the white part from the chive |

**Sauce ingredients**

| | |
|---|---|
| ⅓ cup | orange juice concentrate |
| 2 Tbsp. | oyster sauce |
| 1 Tbsp. | sesame oil |
| 1 Tbsp. | rice vinegar |
| 1 Tbsp. | cornstarch |
| 1 tsp. | chili sauce or 1 Tbsp. dried red pepper flakes |
| | salt and pepper to taste |
| 1 cup | peanuts, unsalted, dry-roasted |

1. Prepare sauce ingredients, set aside.
2. Heat oil in skillet. Add garlic, ginger and onions. Stir-fry for 30 seconds. Add chicken, and stir-fry 4–5 minutes or until cooked through.
3. Stir sauce ingredients together in a small bowl and pour into skillet. Add peanuts and stir until sauce thickens. Adjust seasonings and serve over brown rice. Makes approximately 4 cups.

## Herb-Marinated Chicken Breast

165 calories per 4oz. serving

**Marinade**

| | |
|---|---|
| | zest of 1 lemon |
| | juice of 2 lemons, about ½ cup |
| ¼ cup | olive oil |
| 1 Tbsp. | minced, fresh parsley or 1 tsp. dried |
| 1 Tbsp. | minced, fresh thyme or 1 tsp. dried |
| 1 tsp. | dried dill |
| 1 tsp. | minced garlic |
| | salt and pepper to taste |
| 1½ lbs. | boneless, skinless chicken breasts |

1. Combine all marinade ingredients together in a large resealable bag. Add chicken and marinate overnight.
2. To bake, place chicken on baking sheet sprayed with non-stick cooking spray. Discard marinade. Bake chicken at 350° F for approximately 20 minutes or until chicken is cooked through. Serves 4.

## Chicken Paprika

235 calories per ¼-cup serving

| | |
|---|---|
| 2 Tbsp. | **olive oil** |
| 1 Tbsp. | **minced garlic** |
| 2 | **onions, chopped** |
| 1 lb. | **boneless, skinless chicken breasts, cut into bite-size chunks** |
| 2 | **green bell peppers, chopped** |
| | **salt and pepper** |
| 3 | **Tbsp. tomato paste** |
| 1 Tbsp. | **Hungarian paprika (regular paprika can substitute)** |

1. Heat oil in skillet. Add garlic and onion; stir-fry 4–5 minutes. Add chicken and cook until meat is cooked through, approximately 5 minutes. Add remaining ingredients, and stir to combine and warm through. Serves 4 (¾-cup) servings.

## Chicken Kabobs with Vegetables

178 calories for 2 kabobs

| | |
|---|---|
| 1 lb. | **boneless, skinless chicken breasts cut into small cubes** |
| 1 pint | **cherry tomatoes** |
| 1 pint | **button mushrooms** |
| 1 | **green bell pepper, cut into large chunks** |
| 1 | **red bell pepper, cut into large chunks** |
| 1 | **red or white onion, cut into large chunks** |

**Marinade**

| | |
|---|---|
| ½ cup | **lemon juice** |
| ½ cup | **olive oil** |
| 1 tsp. | **salt** |
| 1 tsp. | **pepper** |
| 1 tsp. | **minced garlic** |
| 1 | **onion, quartered** |
| 1 Tbsp. | **minced, fresh thyme or 1 tsp. dried** |

1. Prepare all meat and vegetables. Combine marinade ingredients. Toss meat and vegetables in marinade and let marinate 2–3 hours.
2. Alternating vegetable and meat, thread onto metal skewers. Grill or broil 10 minutes or until chicken is cooked through. Makes 10 skewers.

## Chicken Puttanesca

320 calories for 1 chicken breast and ½ cup pasta

| | |
|---|---|
| 1 Tbsp. | **olive oil** |
| 6 | **boneless, skinless chicken breasts (approximately 2½ lbs.)** |
| 1 medium | **onion, chopped** |
| 2 Tbsp. | **minced garlic** |
| 12 | **Roma tomatoes (2 lbs.) peeled and chopped, or 2 (28-oz.) cans diced tomatoes** |
| ¼ cup | **balsamic vinegar** |
| 1 Tbsp. | **drained capers** |
| 8–10 | **black or green olives, thinly sliced** |
| 1 Tbsp. | **minced, rinsed anchovies** |
| | **salt and freshly ground black pepper** |
| ¼ tsp. | **crushed red peppers** |
| 1 lb. | **whole-wheat linguine** |

1. Heat olive oil in large skillet over medium high heat. Add chicken and cook 3–4 minutes until lightly browned. Remove from pan and set aside.
2. Add onion and garlic. Sauté 2–3 minutes.
3. Add tomatoes, wine, vinegar, capers, olives and anchovies. Simmer uncovered for 5 minutes, stirring often. Adjust seasonings. Add reserved chicken breasts, making sure they are covered in sauce. Simmer uncovered for 5–10 minutes, or until chicken is cooked through.
4. Meanwhile, bring a large pot of salted water to a boil. Cook pasta 7–10 minutes. Drain, toss and place on large serving platter. Place chicken on top and drizzle with sauce. Serves 6.

## Steamed or Broiled Halibut

245 calories per 6-oz. serving

| | |
|---|---|
| 4 (8-oz.) | **halibut fillets** |
| 2 Tbsp. | **minced, fresh ginger** |
| | **lemon slices and wedges** |

1. Place halibut on steamer rack; if you don't have a steamer, place halibut on a baking sheet sprayed with non-stick cooking spray. Top with ginger and lemon. Place in steamer over boiling water, and steam for approximately 12 minutes or until fish flakes easily. (Or broil 6" under broiler for 10–12 minutes).
2. When fish is done, remove to serving platter and serve with additional lemon wedges. Makes 4 (6-oz.) cooked fillets.

## Balsamic-Glazed Steamed Fish

260 calories per 6-oz. serving

| | |
|---|---|
| 4 (8-oz.) | **fish fillets of choice** |
| ¼ cup | **fat-free chicken broth** |
| 1 Tbsp. | **balsamic vinegar** |
| 1 Tbsp. | **soy sauce** |
| ½ tsp. | **cornstarch** |
| 2 | **green onions, minced** |

1. Place fish fillets on steamer rack over boiling water. Sprinkle fish with salt and pepper. Cover and steam approximately 10 minutes per inch, or bake at 375° F until fish flakes easily.
2. Combine broth, vinegar, sugar, soy sauce and cornstarch in a small saucepan. Bring to a boil; cook until sauce thickens. Remove from heat. Spoon glaze over fish; top with green onion. Makes 4 (6-oz.) cooked servings of fish.

## Whole Baked Salmon with Spicy Apricot Glaze

350 calories per 6-oz. erving

| | |
|---|---|
| 2–3 lbs. | **whole salmon, cleaned** |
| 2 | **lemons, cut into wedges** |
| | **ginger root cut into julienne strips several large sprigs of fresh dill, or 1 Tbsp. dried** |

1. Spray baking sheet with non-stick spray. Place salmon on baking sheet. Layer lemon slices, ginger root and dill in the center cavity of salmon. Loosely cover with foil and bake at 350° F for approximately 30–40 minutes or until fish flakes easily with a fork.
2. Meanwhile, prepare sauce. Recipe follows.
3. When salmon is cooked through, serve with sauce and fresh lemon wedges.

Serve in 6-oz. portions.
(2 lbs. fish=4 portions, 3 lbs. fish=6 portions)

*If you want to use salmon fillets instead of whole salmon, you may (8-oz. fillet=6 oz. cooked). Lay seasonings on top of each fillet and cook in the same manner for about 15 minutes or until cooked through.

## Spicy Apricot Glaze

| | |
|---|---|
| 3 | **shallots, minced** |
| 1 tsp. | **olive oil** |
| 2 Tbsp. | **soy sauce** |
| ½ cup | **apricot jam** |
| 1 Tbsp. | **minced ginger root** |
| 1 tsp. | **minced garlic** |
| 1 Tbsp. | **lime or lemon juice** |
| 1 tsp. | **zest of lime or lemon (optional)** |

1. Heat skillet and sauté shallots in oil for 1–2 minutes. Stir in remaining ingredients. Simmer to warm through. Makes about ¾ cup.

## Grilled, Marinated London Broil

260 calories per 4-oz. serving

| | |
|---|---|
| 2 lbs. | **lean London broil, thinly sliced (flank steak may be substituted)** |

**Marinade**

| | |
|---|---|
| 1½ cups | **soy sauce** |
| ¾ cup | **rice vinegar** |
| ¾ cup | **sherry or cooking sherry** |
| 2 tsp. | **Chinese five spice (or substitute with ½ tsp. each, nutmeg, ginger and cloves, and 1 whole star anise)** |
| 1" piece | **ginger root** |
| ⅓ cup | **sugar** |

1. Combine all marinade ingredients in a large bowl. Place meat in marinade, cover and let set 8 hours. Turn meat in marinade 2 or 3 times during the 8-hour period.
2. Heat grill to medium high. Grill for only 2–3 minutes on each side. Makes 6 (4-oz.) cooked servings.

## Lasagna

320 calories per 2"x4" piece

| | |
|---|---|
| ½ lb. | **lean ground beef** |
| 1 | **onion, chopped** |
| 1 (28-oz.) jar | **spaghetti sauce** |
| 12 | **lasagna noodles** |
| 1 cup | **shredded part-skim mozzarella cheese** |
| 15 oz. | **non-fat ricotta cheese** |
| ¼ cup | **Parmesan cheese** |

1. In large skillet, brown meat with onion and drain off fat. Stir in spaghetti sauce; set aside.
2. Spread a small amount of sauce in the bottom of a baking dish.
3. Arrange one layer of uncooked lasagna noodles over sauce.
4. Stir mozzarella and ricotta cheese together in a small bowl. Spread a thin layer over noodles.
5. Pour a layer of meat sauce over cheese and continue this pattern.
6. Sprinkle with Parmesan cheese. Cover with foil and bake at 350º F for 45 minutes.
7. Remove foil and bake 10 minutes more. Let stand 10 minutes before serving. Serves 4–6.

## Lemon Halibut

245 calories per 6-oz. serving

| | |
|---|---|
| 4 (8-oz.) | **halibut fillets** |
| 2 Tbsp. | **minced, fresh ginger** |
| | **lemon slices and wedges** |

Place halibut on a baking sheet sprayed with non-stick cooking spray. Top with ginger and lemon. Broil 6" under broiler for 10–12 minutes or until done. Serve with additional lemon wedges, if desired. Makes 4 (6-oz.) cooked fillets.

## Beef or Chicken Stew

220 calories per 1-cup serving

| | |
|---|---|
| 1 lb. | **beef stew meat** |
| 1 | **onion, chopped** |
| 3 large | **carrots, diced** |
| 2 | **russet potatoes, diced** |
| 2 cups | **tomato juice or Spicy V-8® juice** |
| 1 (15-oz.) can | **low-fat beef broth** |
| | **salt and pepper to taste** |

Place all ingredients in oven-safe pot. Cover and bake at 350º F for 2½–3 hours until meat is tender. Serves 4.

## Chef Salad

280 calories per 3-cup serving

| | |
|---|---|
| 2 10-oz. bags | **dark, leafy green salad mix** |
| 2 cups | **chopped vegetables of choice** |
| 3 cups | **precooked, chopped chicken, turkey or lean ham (from deli)** |
| 4 | **boiled eggs** |
| ½ cup | **part-skim mozzarella cheese** |

Toss all ingredients together and serve with low-fat salad dressing. Serves 4.

## Chili

220 calories per 1-cup serving

| | |
|---|---|
| 2 (15-oz.) cans | **red kidney beans, drained** |
| 2 (14-oz.) cans | **diced or crushed, tomatoes** |
| 1/2 lb. | **lean ground beef, browned (optional)** |
| 1 | **onion, chopped** |
| 1 package | **chili seasoning mix (or 1 tsp. minced garlic, 2 Tbsp. chili powder, 1 tsp. salt and pepper, 1 tsp. red pepper, and 1 tsp. cumin)** |

Combine all ingredients in a large soup pot. Heat to boiling, reduce and simmer 15 minutes to an hour. Serves 4.

## Sloppy Joes

300 calories per ½-cup serving (includes whole-wheat bun)

| | |
|---|---|
| 1 lb. | **extra-lean ground beef or ground turkey** |
| 1 packet | **sloppy joe seasoning** |
| 1 (6-oz.) can | **tomato paste** |
| 1 package | **whole-wheat buns** |

Prepare according to directions on seasoning packet. Serves 4.

## Stir-fry with Chicken or Shrimp

300 calories per 2-cup serving

| | |
|---|---|
| 1 (28-oz.) bag | **Frozen Vegetable Stir-Fry** |
| 1 lb. | **boneless, skinless chicken breasts or precooked shrimp** |
| 1 Tbsp. | **canola or olive oil** |

Cut chicken into bite-size pieces and stir-fry 3–5 minutes until chicken is cooked through. Add vegetables and cook 5–10 minutes more until veggies are heated through. Season to taste. Serves 4–6.

## Lemon Dill Rice

130 calories per ⅓-cup serving

| | |
|---|---|
| 1 Tbsp. | **olive oil** |
| 1–2 tsp. | **minced garlic** |
| 1–2 tsp. | **minced ginger root** |
| 1 tsp. | **dried dill** |
| 4 cups | **cooked wild rice** |
| | **juice of 1 lemon, about ¼ cup** |
| ⅓ cup | **slivered almonds** |
| | **salt and pepper to taste** |

1. Heat oil in skillet. Add garlic and ginger root and stir-fry 30 seconds. Add remaining ingredients. Heat through and season to taste. Makes approximately 4 cups.

## Seasoned, Boiled Red Potatoes

70 calories per ½-cup serving

| | |
|---|---|
| 1 lb. | **small red potatoes** |
| 1 | **lemon** |
| 1 tsp. | **Italian seasonings** |
| | **salt and pepper** |

1. Cover red potatoes with water and boil approximately 20 minutes, or until tender when pierced with a knife.
2. Drain and season potatoes with the juice of one lemon. Toss with Italian seasonings; salt and pepper to taste. Makes approximately 2½ cups.

## Grilled Vegetables

90 calories per ½-cup serving

| | |
|---|---|
| 1 | **crookneck squash, sliced lengthwise into strips** |
| 1 | **zucchini squash, sliced lengthwise into strips** |
| 2 | **Portabello mushrooms** |
| 1 | **red onion, sliced crosswise into thick rings** |
| 3 Tbsp. | **olive oil** |
| | **salt and pepper** |

1. Place all vegetables on large baking sheet. Drizzle with olive oil, and season with salt and pepper. Stir to coat oil and seasonings over vegetables.
2. Place the vegetables on grill with London broil. The vegetables will cook a few minutes longer than the beef. Makes approximately 3 cups.

## Salsa

25 calories per ½-cup serving

| | |
|---|---|
| 3 | **tomatoes** |
| ¼ | **red onion, minced** |
| ¼ | **bunch fresh cilantro, use less if you like** |
| ½ | **jalapeno, seeds removed and minced** |
| ¼ cup | **lime juice** |
| | **salt and pepper to taste** |

1. Combine all ingredients and serve. Makes about 3 cups.

## Tabbouleh Salad

115 calories per ½-cup serving

| | |
|---|---|
| 1 cup | **cracked wheat bulgar** |
| 2 cups | **boiling water** |
| 2½ Tbsp. | **olive oil** |
| 2½ Tbsp. | **lemon juice** |
| | **salt and pepper to taste** |
| ½ cup | **chopped parsley** |
| ¼ cup | **chopped cilantro** |
| ½ bunch | **minced green onions** |
| 1 large | **tomato, chopped** |
| ¼ cup | **diced celery** |
| ½ | **cucumber, diced** |

1. Pour boiling water over bulgar wheat in bowl. Let stand 1 hour. Meanwhile, prepare all other ingredients. When liquid is absorbed, grain is ready. Add remaining ingredients and stir well. Serve cold. Makes approximately 41/2 cups.

## Citrus Pasta Salad

125 calories per 1-cup serving

| | |
|---|---|
| 3 oz. | **favorite pasta (preferably whole-grain; try bow tie, fusilli, rotelli) cooked according to package directions** |
| 1½ | **oranges, segmented and cut into bite-size pieces** |
| ⅓ cup | **each green and red grapes** |
| ½ (15-oz.) can | **garbanzo beans, drained** |
| ¼ cup | **each broccoli and cauliflower florets** |
| 1½ | **green onions minced** |

**Dressing**

| | |
|---|---|
| 2 Tbsp. | **red wine vinegar, or red wine rosemary vinegar** |
| 2½ Tbsp. | **orange juice concentrate** |
| 1 Tbsp. | **each, fresh basil and oregano, minced, or ½ tsp. each, dried** |
| ¼ tsp. | **minced garlic** |
| | **salt and pepper to taste** |

1. Combine all salad ingredients in a large bowl; toss together well. Mix dressing ingredients together in a small bowl, pour over salad. Cover and chill at least one hour, stirring occasionally. Makes approximately 5 cups.

# Tips for Eating Away from Home

## Italian Food

- Think red and green. Go for red sauces and avoid creamy, fat-laden white sauces. Green means salad; it goes great with any Italian dish.

- Enjoy one or two breadsticks but no more. (This one is hard for me.) If you load up on bread, order soup and a salad and forget the pasta.

- Italian dessert is so temping! Skip it. Some desserts can pack more calories than your entire meal. If you must indulge, share with other people. Try sorbet or fruit ice. Once in a while (like a few times a year), go ahead and enjoy.

- Pasta is infamous for being served in large portions. Try to eat half and save the rest for later.

- Skip stuffed pizzas and calzones.

- Get a little saucy! Ask for half the cheese on your pizza.

## Mexican Food

- Ask for corn tortillas instead of flour tortillas.

- Skip fried taco shells; ask for a soft shell.

- Be careful with taco salads. If you top it with full-fat salad dressing, ask for no guacamole or sour cream. Your best bet is to enjoy the healthy–fat-based guacamole as your dressing.

- Save yourself from nachos or "grande" nachos.

- Ask for black beans instead of refried beans.

- Enjoy salsa as a salad dressing. Or enjoy salsa with a torn-up warm tortilla instead of loading up on chips.

- Fajitas can be a great choice, but skip the side order of rice. The beans and tortillas provide all the carbohydrates you need. Also try to enjoy two fajitas instead of four or five. (Again, take the rest home.)

- Go for "one" instead of "two." Many times, Mexican entrees come with two of everything, "two enchiladas" or "two tacos." Enjoy one entrée with a salad or black beans instead.

## Steak and Seafood

- Go easy on breaded and fried seafood. If you must order fried shrimp (my husband's all-time favorite) then balance your meal with steamed vegetables or salad instead of more fried food (like french fries or onion rings).
- Skip huge chef or Caesar salads. If you order Caesar salad, ask for your dressing on the side.
- Skip loaded baked potatoes. Instead, enjoy half a baked potato with salt and pepper or just one of the offending toppings (butter, sour cream, cheese, or bacon).
- If the restaurant offers endless warm bread, enjoy one serving. If you must load up on bread, order a salad and possibly soup and be done.
- Trim all visible fat from your meat. Not only will you save yourself extra calories, but you will also avoid gnawing on straight gristle.
- Order grilled chicken, broiled fish, filet mignon without the bacon.
- Skip the porterhouse, prime rib, baby-back ribs, T-bone steaks, and meat pies.
- Try to keep portions of meat to eight ounces or less.

## Chinese Food

- Order steamed rice instead of fried rice.
- Go for entrées that include vegetables, like "beef with broccoli" or "chicken with string beans."
- Skip the egg rolls.
- Try to order one entrée instead of two or three. Chinese restaurants are great at marketing combination platters.
- Order entrées with chicken, shrimp, or lean beef instead of duck, spare ribs, or pork.
- Go for "hot and spicy" instead of "sweet and sour" or "crispy" dishes.

## Fast Food and Sandwiches

- Skip french fries. Have a hamburger with a salad or even fresh fruit, like a banana or an apple. (Fresh fruit is easily totable in your car or office; you should always keep some on hand.)

- Order grilled chicken or small hamburgers. Yes, this means skip the double, triple, or half-pound burgers.

- Skip shakes. A 16-ounce vanilla shake can easily have more than 430 calories, which can burst anyone's calorie budget. Enjoy a shake once in a while as a snack or stand-alone item but not with an already calorie-packed meal.

- Enjoy baked potatoes when offered.

- For kids, go for fruit slices and milk instead of soda pop and french fries.

- Enjoy just one slice of pizza at fast-food pizza outlets.

- Sandwiches are a great choice, but think small, no more than six inches long (unless you order a low-fat veggie or meat-and-veggie sandwich with no mayo or cheese). Choose whole-grain breads and plenty of veggies.

- Remember that adding mayo and cheese to a sandwich will tack on another 200 calories, at least.

- Don't be fooled by a grilled-cheese sandwich. It may seem small and simple, but the thick filling of cheese and buttered white bread slyly serves up a good 600 calories.

- Order baked chips or enjoy fruit as a side item for sandwiches.

## Breakfast Food

- Order fruit, yogurt, milk, or small servings of whole-grain breads and cereals whenever possible.

- Use jam instead of cream cheese.

- Try a whole-grain cereal bar.

- Top a waffle with fruit instead of syrup. Or try reduced-calorie syrup.

- Try cottage cheese and fruit.

- Avoid having dessert for breakfast—chocolate donuts with candy sprinkles, chocolate or cookie cereals, or high-sugar fruit drinks.

- Skip the fatty meats and sweets—sausage, bacon, giant cinnamon rolls, toppling muffins, or Danish pastries and donuts.

- If you enjoy eating meat at breakfast, go for lean ham or turkey, egg substitutes, or, a few times per week, whole cooked eggs.

- Skip loaded omelettes with cheese and meat. Instead, try scrambled eggs with salsa or peppers.

- For a healthy dine-in breakfast, your absolute best option is hot or cold whole-grain cereal (like oatmeal), scrambled eggs (or egg substitute), and fruit.

## Mall and Airport Food

- Order plain pretzels instead of buttery pretzels with a rich dipping sauce.

- Try a small fruit smoothie as a snack or a quick breakfast.

- Order a salad as your main dish.

- Instead of ice cream, try frozen yogurt or sorbet.

- If you can't resist temptation, then once in a while (and no, that does not mean every week) enjoy a small cookie, half of a cinnamon roll (share it, please!), or a small serving of your favorite ice cream. But don't make these items a regular part of your diet.

- If you decide to go for a dish of ice cream, go easy on the topping. Stick with fresh fruit or nuts. Adding something as simple as hot fudge and candy sprinkles can turn a dish of ice cream into a treat that packs as many calories as a decent meal.

# Questions and Answers

*Q: Should I limit carbohydrates, use low-carbohydrate foods, or try a low-carb diet?*

A: Of all the carbohydrate foods we consume, the large muffins, refined cereals and breads, giant cinnamon rolls, and platters of pasta are the foods we consume in excess. So go ahead—limit refined, processed, oversized carbohydrate foods. But don't limit healthy whole grains, fruits, vegetables, and low-fat dairy products (which are all sources of carbohydrates). Low-carbohydrate foods are expensive and unnecessary. Sometimes products labeled "low carb" have more fat and essentially more calories than their original carbohydrate counterpart.

Carbohydrates are the main source of fuel for the body, and not just for activity. Carbohydrates provide the fuel for your lungs to breathe, your heart to pump, and your brain to function. Low-carb diets essentially "trick" your metabolism into losing weight. And tricking your metabolism is not something you can do for a lifetime. Second, low-carbohydrate diets restrict the foods that protect our health—whole grains, fruits, and vegetables—and vamp up foods we know to be detrimental in large amounts—fat, saturated fat, cholesterol, and sodium. Finally, these diets don't fit with the Word of Wisdom. Read Doctrine and Covenants section 89, pray about it, ponder it, and then see what your heart tells you.

*Q: Should I limit salt intake?*

A: The National Committee on Prevention, Evaluation, and Treatment of High Blood Pressure recommends that we consume no more than 2,400 milligrams of sodium per day. The most recent data (1999–2000) from the National Health and Examination Survey show that the average intake of sodium in the United States is approximately 3,400 milligrams per day. A plethora of research has linked high sodium consumption to high blood pressure. However, we know that only a percentage of us are "salt sensitive." The term "salt sensitive" means that blood pressure rises in response to high sodium intake or, conversely, decreases with sodium restriction. Approximately 50 percent of the people with diagnosed hypertension and 25 percent of people without hypertension are classified as salt sensitive.[1]

The bottom line is yes, you should be concerned about salt because we consume too much. However, because of the salt sensitivity of certain people, cutting back on salt doesn't always guarantee better control of high blood pressure. Regardless, we need to cut back on processed and fast foods, cut back on adding salt to food during cooking and at the table, and choose more reduced-sodium products.

*Q: Should I be concerned about sugar?*

A: A 20-ounce bottle of soda pop has almost 17 teaspoons of sugar. A 44-ounce fountain beverage (non-diet) has more than 36 teaspoons of sugar! A normal one and a half cup serving of sweetened cereal has 6 teaspoons of sugar. The best part the USDA recommends that we consume no more than 10 teaspoons of sugar per day.

The answer is yes, we should be concerned about sugar. But if you stick to the advice in this book most of the time (a good 80 to 90 percent of the time), you will be just fine. Make it a point to limit sugary beverages (soda, juice, lemonade, fruit drinks), candy, sweetened cereals, ice cream, and other sweet treats.

*Q: Are artificial sweeteners (sugar substitutes) safe?*

A: Of all the artificial sweeteners on the market, sucralose (or Splenda®) seems to be the safest. It works great in cooking and can easily be substituted cup for cup. The other popular substitute, aspartame (also known as Equal®, NutraSweet®, or NutraTaste) is probably safe, but certain people with a rare disorder called phenylketonuria (PKU) should avoid aspartame completely. Aspartame is made from two amino acids, aspartic acid and phenylalanine. Some people believe aspartame to be the cause of everything from headaches to multiple sclerosis to Alzheimer's disease. There is no scientific evidence to back up such claims. Besides, the human body is not that generic. One single compound is not the cause of all human ailments and diseases.

Anything used in excess can be unhealthful for our bodies. Personally, I do use sugar substitutes but try hard to do so in moderation. I prefer to use a sugar substitute in foods that are normally very high in sugar, such as beverages, maple syrup, or baked goods. I also use sugar substitutes to sweeten some cereals or desserts. Otherwise, I just go for a small serving of the real thing.

*Q: Should I take a nutritional supplement?*

A: Since 90 percent of us have a diet that is "poor" or "needs improvement," then at least 90 percent of us should take a multivitamin/mineral supplement. Many of us have eating habits that are monotonous and at the same time unpredictable. Many of us, try as we may, just don't get enough of the vitamin-packed fruits and vegetables we need every day. A vitamin/mineral supplement can provide the little extra support we need. You don't have to spend a lot of money to get a good multivitamin/mineral supplement. Simply look for a brand that supplies you with 100 percent or less of the RDA for each nutrient. Remember, we also get nutrients from food, so in most circumstances 100 percent or less of the RDA is perfectly appropriate. Some nutrients are water soluble and not stored by the body, so extra amounts are simply excreted in the urine. On the other hand, some nutrients are fat soluble and stored by the body, and too much can be toxic. If you choose to "load up" on any particular vitamin or mineral, you should check with your physician before doing so.

*Q: What about diet bars and shakes?*

A: If you find yourself in a "must-have-chocolate" crunch and your choice is a bag of Oreos or a chocolate-covered diet bar, go for the diet bar. Diet or protein bars and shakes really can be part of a healthful diet, and they can be quite helpful during busy times. I recommend Clif bars, Luna bars, Powerbar®, Pria® bars, or Kashi® bars. Several bars on the market are nutritionally equivalent to a candy bar, but if they help you keep your calorie budget intact, then go for it. Of course, fresh fruit or veggies always make a superior snack, but realistically we don't always have access to them. Also, becoming dependent on diet bars and shakes can be detrimental, because when you go back to eating real food, which of course you will, you will have a hard time maintaining your weight. The best way to use these types of food is in moderation.

*Q: What is a safe and maintainable weight-loss goal?*

A: One to two pounds per week is realistic, sensible, safe, and most important, maintainable. Diet programs that promise "10 pounds in a week" or rapid weight loss are playing an unfair and untruthful game with your personal health.

*Q: What if I had a bad week? Is it really worth it to start over—again?*

A: Any attempt to take a step forward for your health is worth it. You can start over at any time. The important thing is to stay on the right path and keep moving forward. It doesn't matter how fast or how slow you progress; what matters is that you are headed in the right direction.

*Q: What if my kids refuse to eat healthy?*

A: All kids go through picky phases. My children are toddlers, and "picky" doesn't even begin to describe their eating habits. I have to play all kinds of games with my kids. Green beans are snakes; broccoli florets are trees; grapes come in "mommy," "daddy," and "baby" sizes; casseroles are dropped onto dinner plates in the shapes of A's and B's; and milk makes our bones strong (okay, so I may also have said that little girls' bones can crack like the dinosaurs' bones did if we don't drink enough milk; does lying for health reasons really count as a lie?).

You also have to be patient with kids. You may have to introduce new foods several times before they finally accept them. But the important thing is to keep offering healthy foods. Your kids will come around. Cut up fresh fruit or serve up veggies and dip for an after-school snack. Keep healthy foods visible. Keep the unhealthy foods invisible, or better yet, out of the house completely. Kids need to learn to eat healthy, and they need to see you eating healthy as a good example. Don't make your kids clean their plates. Let them learn to listen to their own hunger cues; allow them to eat when they are hungry and stop when they are full. If the kids are begging for food right before dinner or another meal, tide them over with something healthful. Most of all, don't ever use food as a reward or a punishment. Kids need to understand that food is part of everyday normal living and not something to be hoarded or shunned.

*Q: How can I get my children to be more active?*

A: Allow only one to two hours per day on the computer, playing video games, or watching TV. Kids can start doing things like running, playing games, riding bikes, going for hikes, doing aerobics with Mom, or even playing sports at a very young age. Make sure your kids have some sort of physical activity every day; their growing bodies need physical activity to develop strong muscles and bones and a healthy metabolism. Nobody is doing their children any favors by allowing them to engage in a sedentary lifestyle. In November of 2003, at the American Academy of Pediatrics' annual meeting, our U.S. Surgeon General said this: "Our children deserve much better than a lifetime of expensive and potentially fatal medical complications associated with excess weight." If your children refuse to get moving, help them find a sport or activity they enjoy. It may take a few tries, but the rewards will pay off for a lifetime.

*Q: Should I exercise in the morning or evening?*

A: This one is easy: whenever you can stick to it. However, I usually urge morning workouts, whether inconvenient or not, because too many things come up during the day that get in the way of our valiant attempts to exercise. Some people do really well with an evening exercise routine. However, most people, by the time evening rolls around, find that energy levels are at rock-bottom lows and exhaustion has overtaken any well-intended goals to exercise.

*Q: Is it bad to eat after 8:00 P.M.?*

A: Not necessarily. Your metabolism doesn't suddenly change into "store everything as fat" mode after a certain hour of the day. Rather, later in the evening is when most of us indulge in higher-fat and higher-calorie foods. This is the time of day when we are more likely to chow down on a pint of ice cream, mindlessly eat an entire bag of popcorn, or munch on other salty and sweet treats. Eating later in the evening can also be a problem because we don't burn a lot of calories sleeping. That is why you should eat a good breakfast and lunch—you will be moving throughout the day and using those calories. People who skip breakfast and often lunch and then devour a heavy dinner are prone to have weight-control problems. Set a goal to eat several small meals and snacks throughout the day. In other words, eat less, more often.

# Testimonials

## Michael Ballam

It is hard to believe the difference the Losing It! exercise and fitness program brought into my life. I was on the brink of despair about my physical condition. I had given up hope of ever having a better quality of life. At the age of 53, as the CEO of a high-stress multimillion dollar company, I had resigned myself to always feeling lethargic, lacking in energy, and destined to spend what should be my most productive years dragging myself to and from work. The pounds kept piling on, and the energy and optimism kept evaporating away. I was up to 209 pounds, which on my modest frame of 5' 10" slowed me down to a snail's pace. When Monica at ICON did an assessment test, my body fat content was 28.6, my waist measurement was 43.5" (above the navel) and 42.5" (at the navel) and 40"

(2 inches below), and I was not surprised because I was constantly buying new clothes, which soon became ill fitting and uncomfortable. I was not morbidly obese, but the added pounds and inches made me drag through the day and changed my outlook on life immensely. My personal health was at an all-time low. High cholesterol, high blood pressure, light-headedness, aches and pains, and constant fatigue were plaguing me daily. There is a history of diabetes in our family, and the treat of developing a chronic disease such as that loomed on the horizon. My emotional health was, needless to say, at a low ebb. Having been a very active person, I was resigning myself to feeling ill and nonproductive for the rest of my life.

My blood pressure was often around 150/100, even with diuretics and blood-pressure medication, and my pulse hovered around 90 in a resting state. I was wearing myself out doing *nothing!* I had witnessed a transformation with a colleague of mine who went to ICON for help, and through some gentle and not so gentle urging from family members I walked into ICON's bright, clean, upbeat facility for a day that would change my life for the better. I have had memberships at health clubs but fell into activity because I was uncomfortable with some of the elements there: namely, the physical merchandising (over-achieving clients who take up residence in the gym to preen and pick up other clients). That was a real turn-off for me and made me uncomfortable to attend. In addition, I felt guilty and uncomfortable taking the time of a personal trainer to stand over me time after time to see that I was doing the exercises properly. Both of those elements were eliminated with the Losing It! program.

A personal trainer took all my health history, which is complex and challenging, and provided us with wonderful meal programs where a great deal of latitude of choice is given. There is no magical ingredient about the meal plans (not high carb/low carb, high fat/low fat craziness)—just nutritional meals, being aware of calorie intake through three balanced meals and snacks. I actually found it interesting to become more in control of what foods brought the most enjoyment and energy without compounding calories and weight gain.

Within three weeks I dropped 24 pounds. What a difference it made in the way I felt! I had energy all through the day and particularly at night, when before I was always watching the clock, hoping bedtime would soon come to pass. The entire workout program could be enacted in just over an hour, and I gained 3 hours of productivity during the day. That is quite a payoff! I am truly converted and don't want to go back to the way I was. This program really works, and the people at ICON know what they are doing!

## Kent Ware

I was diagnosed with Type II diabetes over ten years ago. I take insulin and an oral medication. I work in an office, am a little over 50 years old, and am about 15 pounds over my ideal weight. For years I've had a desire to be a little more active, have better control over my blood-sugar levels, and lose those extra pounds. Sure, I've made goals and set up programs and diets to follow, but they have all been short lived.

I was at the point where I was telling myself it was time to try again when I learned that Melanie Douglass was introducing a health and fitness plan to the associates in our company. I attended the kick-off meeting and picked up the materials. What impressed me most was that the program was simple, easy to understand, and flexible. I didn't want to go on another diet or exercise plan; I wanted to make a lifestyle change. This seemed to be the plan that could help me do that. I made a commitment to follow it for 13 weeks.

The goals I set centered around general health and activity. I did not have a specific weight-loss goal. Rather, my goal was to follow the eating and exercise plan at least five days a week. The meal plan included a 400-calorie breakfast, 400-calorie lunch, 500-calorie dinner, and 600 calories of optional snacks. The activity plan included 30 minutes a day of an aerobic activity alternated with a 30-minute strength-training workout on alternating days. Both plans were easy to understand from the materials provided. My objective was not to complete the 13 weeks and then stop. I wanted to make a lifestyle change.

The results of the 13-week program for me are as follows:

1. I was successful at following the plan six days per week (one more day per week than my initial commitment).

2. My blood-sugar scores improved by about 25 percent. I am now within the 70–140 range almost every time I test.

3. My insulin use dropped by 33 percent. (This happened within the first two weeks and has stayed down since.)

4. My HgbA1c score dropped from 7.9 to 7.5 percent. (It has never before been that low.)

5. My lipid profile improved several points in every category.

6. My weight dropped from 188 to 175 pounds (1 pound per week on average).

7. I lost two inches from my waist (from size 36 to 34).

8. My energy level has improved, and I feel better about myself.

Some things I especially like about this program:

1. It was flexible. I determined the fitness goals that were most important to me.

2. The calorie approach was easier for me to manage than counting carbohydrates (which I had been taught to do as a diabetic).

3. The meal suggestions (including those for eating out) were easy to follow and fit in with today's active lifestyles. They included easy-to-prepare and off-the-shelf foods—not to mention the fast-food and restaurant recommendations.

4. The fitness plan using the ball and weights was easy to follow. The instructions were clear and detailed (including breathing). It gave me a good workout without exhausting me.

5. It was helpful to be doing this as part of a group of associates. It was important that I was asked to share my goal with a person who I knew would be checking back with me in 6 and 13 weeks for accountability. I knew there would be a time when I could raise my

hand in a company meeting to signify that I had accomplished my goal. (It was also help-ful that the president of the company had offered an incentive for those who met their health and fitness goal.)

Some things I did that made the program more successful for me personally:

1. I shared my goals and commitment with my family at home.

2. I created a log book with sections where I could record my fitness activity, meals, snacks, blood-sugar scores, and insulin use for every day. Each page represented a week. My goal was printed at the top of the page for easy reference. I included a box that I would check each time I accomplished a specific goal. There was a box at the top of the page that I would check when I met my goal for the week. The log became not only a place to track my progress but also a personal accountability tool. I put the pages in a three-ring binder so the active week was the first page with previous weeks behind it, followed by the fitness instructions, meal suggestions, and calorie charts. I took the binder to work during the day and kept it by my desk for easy access. At night I kept it next to my glucometer. Checking off the "goal accomplished" boxes throughout the day and recording events as they occurred made a big difference in sticking with the program.

3. I made fitness a priority. In the past I've tried getting up early in the morning to exercise. (I usually have more energy in the morning.) But it doesn't take long before a couple of late nights in a row make it too easy to hit the snooze button and sleep the extra half hour. This time I decided I would exercise the first 30 minutes after arriving home from work. This is usually when I'm at my tiredest, but I committed to myself that I wouldn't eat dinner until I'd exercised. (Eating is enough of a reward for me that it was a good motivator.) I found that the exercising improved my energy level for the rest of the evening and suppressed my appetite so I felt fuller and more satisfied with less food.

4. I checked my weight only once a week. Checking more often only emphasizes that progress is slow and makes things more discouraging. Besides, for me, losing weight was

not the goal. I knew if I ate better and increased my activity I was likely to lose some weight, but I didn't make it a goal because I didn't want to get discouraged if it didn't reach a specific weight goal.

5. I set goals I was fairly confident I could reach . . . and then I set out to beat them. I know myself well enough to know that I get a charge out of not just meeting a deadline but beating it. I assumed the same would be true with this program. They recommended following the meal and fitness plan six days a week. I set a goal to do it five days a week, knowing that I would feel better about myself when I "beat" my goal by doing it six days a week. I also knew that if I set my goal at six days a week and missed on one day, it would discourage me enough to make me want to just give up altogether. It really worked. There were two weeks where I only "met" my goal. That didn't discourage me. It only made me want to try harder to "beat" my goal the next week.

The good news is that now, three to four months after completing the plan, I have maintained my weight and waist size, incorporated the principles of the meal planning and calorie counting into my daily routine, and included regular exercise and fitness into my lifestyle. I feel I have the confidence to continue this lifestyle into the future.

## Kathryn Haroldsen

I have struggled with weight my whole life. I would try the latest fad diet and only stick with it for a couple of weeks, and I would exercise but soon quit because I lacked motivation when I did not see results. When I got married, I was at a weight that I felt comfortable with and was happy where I was. But during my first pregnancy, I gained 50 pounds because I thought I could eat what I wanted whenever I wanted and did little exercise. I was only able to lose 30 of those pounds before my second pregnancy, in which I gained 25 pounds. I realized that if I kept this up, my weight would be out of control and I would not be happy with my size. After the birth of my second child, I found that I did not have the energy or the drive to take care of a newborn and chase after my two-and-a-half year old. I was very out of shape and felt bound to the couch as I sent my older child to get things I needed. I was depressed and was not enjoying motherhood. I was not happy with how I looked, and I wanted that to change. I wanted to be healthy.

During this time, my husband was working out at the ICON Fitness Center, which used the Losing It! meal and exercise programs, and he would ask me to go with him. I decided to go and check it out for myself. I was impressed with how the center was set up and how the fitness program illustrated the cardio workout and also the step-by-step instruction for weight lifting. So once I got the okay from my doctor at my six-week check-up, I went into the Fitness Center and got started. I was coming two to three times a week but soon realized that if I really wanted to get in shape I would need to come in five days a week and work even harder. I was gaining a greater appreciation for fitness and for what my body can do, but I needed more knowledge of nutrition and the food that my body needs for fuel. I heard about the 12-week fitness study the ICON Fitness Center was having, and that it involved a nutrition plan along with exercise. I knew it would be a good chance to learn about sensible eating and how to take care of my body's nutritional needs along with the physical needs. I applied and was excited when I was chosen to a part of the study and to see what I could accomplish in reaching my weight loss goal.

I followed the nutrition and exercise plan for the 12 weeks. I enjoyed the food, and I was coming into the Fitness Center four to five days a week, following their exercise program and working out at home. At the end of the 12 weeks I had lost 17 pounds and 12.5 inches and lowered my blood pressure, and my lower-back pain was gone.

From that experience, I have learned that it is important to have daily exercise and also to follow a sensible eating plan. I have continued with what I learned and have lost a total of 30 pounds so far, and I'm still going. I discovered that I got better results when I followed a nutrition plan than just exercising alone. Now I look forward to my workouts and enjoy exercising and the time it allows for myself and to not be mommy for an hour of the day. I definitely have more energy to play with my boys and take care of my home. I am a happier person and have a new passion for life.

## Marc Jensen

*How did I get this fat?*

I know, it sounds like a silly question; after all, I was there when it happened. If anybody should know how it happened, it *should* be me. Yet, few of us are self-cognizant enough to realize why we do what we do when we do it. We just "act." Sometimes we plan ahead, but in day to day life, we just follow the habits and routines that we have developed and can do without thinking. If we are not careful, "fat" is an accident waiting to happen, and, like most accidents, the only way to understand what happened is to review what happened after the fact.

I was not a particularly fat child; few children are, after they get rid of the baby fat and start crawling and walking. That should be the first clue for all of us, but honestly, what toddler thinks, "Hey, I started walking and the baby fat just started dropping off"? No, we aren't aware of the simplest and purest example of action and reaction. Too bad. After all, if we were programmed properly from the beginning, we wouldn't have to go through so much effort later in life.

Let me insert here that every pound of fat I am now fighting to lose I also fought to gain. I didn't realize I was doing so at the time—let's be honest, I enjoyed the pitched battle with those fries, that entire pizza, that second bowl of ice cream—but so often we wonder why we can't lose in weeks what took us *years* to put on.

I had three strikes against me from the beginning: (1) a mother who was an excellent cook and specialized in desserts; (2) those "starving kids in Africa"; and, (3) a more quiet personality. Number 1 is self-explanatory. Number 2 would be as well, but let me comment that I can remember too many times when I was full, with my body saying "enough already," but my taste buds had signed on for an orgy and would not be dissuaded. I took comfort in those poor starving African kids, without ever once considering how my becoming fat would be of benefit to those poor, malnourished malcontents. It was hard-wired into my psyche that I had to clean my plate. It now takes a conscious effort to stop, even when I'm full, even now when I know those starving kids will never benefit if I finish those last few bites.

Number 3 was the last nail in the coffin. I might have survived the first two strikes if I had been an athletic, sports-oriented kid. I wasn't. I love sports . . . on TV . . . with a table filled with snacks. I enjoyed a good book more than a good bike ride. Many are the fond memories of a book, of a day in the library, of a summer reading. And that is where it started.

As I said, I wasn't heavy as a kid. I grew up a half mile from school. A half mile there, a half mile home. A half mile back to play after dinner (school is where we played), and a half mile home. Besides, as a kid you have two means of transportation, feet and a bike. I had both, and I knew how to use them.

When I was nine we moved to another city. School was one block away—an eighth of a mile. Hardly even a stroll. Plus, this was when I learned that a stroll to the library (a quarter of a mile away) would give me hours of reading ("sedentary" was unknown to me at the time, but it was a requirement to read). That is when weight started becoming a problem. It wasn't a big problem. I was "heavy" but still not too bad. After all, I still walked to and from school, and I did have friends I'd go play with.

It got a little worse in high school. Same distance from home, but lives change. Boys go into sports and start dating girls, and those two usually keep them busy enough and active enough, *unless* they prefer books, are not good in sports, and, because they are "heavy," cannot imagine a girl would want to go out with them. Then the vicious cycle starts: (1) I don't want to play/exercise because it is hard *because* I am overweight, so I don't exercise, so I gain more weight, so it is harder to exercise, so I want to do it even less, so I do even less, so I gain more weight, and on and on the spiral. (2) They call me fat, so I will stay home with my books . . . and sulk . . . and eat, because that makes me feel better. I'm sure you can see that spiral as well. Two concurrent spirals, either one of which would add weight but together gang up to beat a poor kid into submission.

Even then I was not terribly "fat" in high school. (I never weighed myself; I didn't want to know, so now I'm not sure how bad I was.) I suspect I was 20 to 30 lbs. overweight, which I'm sure sounds terrible to you people fighting 10 pounds, but for those of us on the spiral that is nothing. It was enough to affect my self-concept, though, but strangely never enough to make me want to change the problem. (This is the other aspect of "How did I get this fat?"; it is gradual enough that you don't realize there is a problem until there is *a problem*.)

After high school I went on a church mission for two years and got into the best shape in my life. I had to cook for myself (actually, I'm a decent cook, so I wasn't starving), but the big difference was that I found myself in the Arizona/California desert—on a bike. I was riding an average of five or more hours a day, in the sun, in 100-degree weather. I actually was, for the first time I could remember, skinny. I was about 145 pounds when I got off my mission (I am 5'8" and "the charts" say I should weigh about 129 to 170 pounds, depending on *which one* you read.)

I went to college and quickly got up to around 175–180 pounds, where I stayed for quite a while. It is about where I felt the best physically. And the nice thing was, I wasn't worrying about my weight at all. I ate what I wanted and didn't think about it. How could that be? In retrospect, I think the thing that saved me was the fact that I lived about a mile from campus. Walk a mile in the morning, a mile in the evening, sometimes make two trips if I had a big break between morning and afternoon classes, and I had learned how to socialize. I was actually too busy to be hungry. I ate, then ran to class. I grabbed something for lunch. I walked home and ate something quick before I ran off to study or the night's activities. If only I'd kept it up.

A few years later, I moved. Instead of being a mile from campus, I was several miles away, and walking was no longer feasible. It didn't seem to be a problem, though; after about six months, my clothes started getting tight, then tighter, and then they didn't fit. Within a year and a half from my moved, I had my first true "How did I get this fat?" moment when I found a scales and weighed in at 245 pounds. Something had to be done, and luckily I was again about to move.

I went on to some postgraduate work at a different university and was "lucky" to find that most apartments near the university were a little too slum-like for my taste. I did find a nice, clean, quiet, "affordable" place about a mile from campus. Surprise, surprise, ten months later I weighed in at 165. I knew by now what the difference was between physical activity and sedentary life, but life doesn't always cooperate.

When I went into "the work force," finding work a mile from home never really worked. The 80 pounds I had lost came back with a vengeance. The "increase," as always, was gradual, but I let it go, and go, and go, until eight years later I topped the scale at 280 pounds. "How did I get this fat?" I knew the answer this time and sought to do something about it. I didn't move; I just forced myself to start walking again. After all, it had always worked before. In five months I was down to 210, but I was depressed. I was walking about two to three hours every day, plus work, plus the commute. Yes, I was losing weight, but all I was doing was working, sleeping, driving, and walking, and it wasn't that exciting of a life. Plus, my feet hurt—a lot—all the time. So I gave up. Quit cold turkey.

In retrospect, it always takes longer to gain it back than lose it, but keeping it off has to be a continual thing. If I quit, it comes back, and always more than before. My most recent "How did I get this fat?" was about two years ago when I found myself in the hospital with deep-vein thrombosis (blood clots). The doctor stuck me in the hospital, telling me, "You could drop over dead any minute if one of those clots breaks loose and hits your lunges." He was delicate about it, but he did mention that one of the factors in my condition was probably my weight. It came back in force: I had hit 350 pounds. Strangely, my feet still hurt, and my back, and most of the rest of me. When you are carrying 200 pounds more than you should, constantly, it wears on you.

I had lost about 22 pounds when I heard of the Losing It! program was offering. My efforts had been haphazard at best, and slow, 22 pounds in six months. I started the program and lost 27 pounds in 12 weeks. It wasn't all that difficult, either. Walk half an hour a day, at a comfortable pace; that I could handle.

The thing that was really eye-opening for me was my caloric intake. I was putting on 1,900 calories a day. At first I thought that would be impossible, but most of the time I was filled at the end of the meals. I wasn't stuffed so I had to waddle away from the table, but I was satisfied. Plus, once a week I could "carefully" let my hair down in my eating.

Most interesting was watching the portions. Over the years I had read or "heard" or was "told" to eat this many ounces, this many calories, one portion, two portions, but seldom could I really understand what the size should be. I don't consider myself particularly dense, but as I read labels or books, calorie counting seemed nearly impossible to figure out—the fact that raw vegetables have a different calorie count than the same amount cooked was just the most obvious "confusion factor." But I watched the portions that were recommended to me of different foods. I could "see" how much pasta, how much fish, how much chicken, what size salad, and the first thing I realized was that I had gotten into the habit of eating two or three portions before I looked for seconds or thirds. I had been so concerned about those starving African kids that I'd been eating enough to feed a small tribe, or at least a large family, daily.

By exercising at least half an hour a day and eating smaller portions, I was able to lose pounds the same way I had in the past, but in the past I could only do it with two or three times the effort and never focusing on my eating habits. I also feel better at the end of a meal—full, not stuffed. And this lifestyle seems workable, something I could do the rest of my life.

Currently I am 60 pounds lighter than I was at my all-time high. That is about a third of what I need to lose to get to where "the charts" say I should be. I feel better physically and can just imagine how much better I will feel when I lose another 100 pounds.

I don't kid myself; I have a weight problem. When I weigh only 175 pounds I will still have a weight problem; it will just be in remission at that point in time. I do know that it is so much easier to just eat sensible portions and exercise half an hour a day—so much easier to keep it off than to lose it. I know *how* to solve the problem and *how* to keep it from ever being a problem again. Now all I have to do is *do it*.

## Susan Oliver

I have been one of the typical people that you have seen and heard of! Any diet, I have tried it! My body has been like a child playing with a balloon, blowing it up and letting it out. Most of my years since the beginnings of motherhood have been spent in the blown-up mode. I spent my younger years spending much time on trying to be the perfect Mother (if there is such a thing) and not spending the time for exercise, watching what I eat, and caring about my weight. I often commented to my husband, "If I could lose weight by the miles I put on the car and how fast the gas pedal would go while running kids here and there, I would be paper thin!" Last summer, when I was down to my last two children at home, I started feeling that I needed to take care of myself a little better. I went to the doctor, and he commented that I had a stressed heart when resting. I emphatically denied it, of course, because I felt great! I had been diagnosed with type-2 diabetes five years before and had been encouraged to lose weight and exercise to maintain my health without having to take the glucaphage I had been prescribed. I went to a cardiologist, of course. After many tests, I found that I was all right. I concluded that I simply *had* to take better care of this earthly temple. I had started to cut back the amounts I had been consuming on my own. I then had the offer from Deseret Book and Sheri Dew. I knew I could do this as I had a good start and had my mind set. I took on this challenge full-bore! I was excited with my feelings about eating, exercise, and most of all my benefits! I was feeling excited about work, family, and life, and I felt a lift in my self-esteem! I love what I am feeling and have still more to lose, and I have enjoyed the compliments from people, but most of all I am thrilled with how I feel. Exercise and food control (I like to call it that as I always want to fight that four-letter word) is an important part of everyday life, just like eating and sleeping. I have a new goal of getting off of my glucaphage eventually. Yes, you too can make a difference in your life! Thank you ICON Health and Deseret Book!

## Paul Mackay

I was recently part of a research study sponsored by ICON Health & Fitness. Before I took part in this study, my lifestyle was as follows:

My wife and I ate out about three to five times a week. If I wasn't eating out with my wife, I was eating fast food at work. I would drink on average 64 to 128 ounces of soda pop a day. On breaks at work I would usually get a treat at the ICON Café. All-in-all my life style was destroying my health.

I started working for ICON about four years ago, and since then I have gained about 40 pounds. I was working out sporadically at work, but I wasn't seeing much success. My doctor had been telling me I need to lose weight, and I knew I needed to make a change, but I wasn't sure how. My doctor told me that just cutting the pop and counting calories would be a good start. When I heard about the research program, I knew this could help me. When I started the program, my weight was 274 pounds, my blood pressure was

136/79, and my resting heart rate was 60 beats per minute. My measurements were 52 inches two inches above my navel, 58 inches at my navel, and 59 inches two inches below my navel. I was really out of shape and in need of a big change in my life.

The program I followed was very simple. I worked out for one hour each day four to five times a week. ICON provided me with meals twice a day, five days a week, for twelve weeks. They helped me determine my daily calories, and the meals followed those caloric recommendations six days a week. I had one free day a week to eat whatever I wanted. Each day I was able to eat 2,100 calories (400 breakfast, 400 lunch, 600 dinner, and 600 bonus). I stopped drinking pop, even diet pop. It was very simple to follow the program. I found that I wasn't very hungry, the further I got into the program. I started to eat less because I wasn't as hungry. The thing I feel that helped me the most was cutting the pop. The pop not only added huge amounts of calories to my diet; it left me feeling bloated. Also, I feel it affected my workouts. I could work out harder after quitting the pop. I could run further without resting. For example, before quitting the pop, I ran about six minutes without stopping. Now I run ten to fifteen minutes without stopping, and I run much faster.

I feel very successful now that I have changed my lifestyle. I eat at home almost every night. If I need to eat out, I go to Subway. At the end of the twelve-week program, my weight was 234 pounds, my blood pressure was 116/71, and my resting heart rate was 48 beats per minute. My measurements were 44 inches two inches above my navel, 44 inches at my navel, and 43 inches two inches below my navel. I lost 40 pounds and a total of 38 inches. That was the week before Thanksgiving. Over the holidays I've lost an additional 10 pounds, and I plan to keep on losing. In conclusion, this wasn't a very hard program to follow. I followed the rules, for the most part. I still had a few bad days, but I stuck to my diet. On my off days, I really blew it, but it didn't have much of an overall effect on my diet.

My results are not atypical; I know others that follow the diet and had similar results.

My wife participated with me and had the same results similar to mine. If you eat healthy foods and follow an exercise program (even walking 20 to 40 minutes a day), you will see results. This is not a "starvation" diet; it *is* an "eat healthy to be healthy" diet.

## Meghan Peterson

My name is Meghan Peterson. I am 15 years old. I've struggled with my weight ever since I was in kindergarten. Every year when I would go up a grade, my weight would go up too. I was not comfortable with how I looked. It was hard for me to do some of the same things that my friends were doing. I loved to dance, but I didn't like the clothes that I had to wear to dance in. When I went into middle school, I was bigger than the girls that were my friends. There were full-length mirrors in the hallways of the middle school, and I hated walking past them. Every time I looked into the mirrors, I saw a girl who was a size I did not want to be. At the end of the seventh-grade, I decided I wanted to do something about being overweight. I had a strong desire to become the size I longed to be and to be able to do things I wasn't able to do because of my size.

That's when I was introduced to a great program and some great people that wanted to help me reach my goal. ICON Health & Fitness were looking at ways they could help youth who had weight problems. They introduced me to Melanie Douglass, a nutritionist, and Heather Guyman, a personal trainer. I loved their program, which was eating healthy and working out. Melanie talked to me about healthy food choices and good proportions. Heather became my personal trainer and good friend. They were very encouraging to me by not making it seem too hard. It was just a better way of life.

I am now more than 70 pounds lighter, and I feel like a new person. I feel so good about myself. Walking past the mirrors at the middle school became something exciting instead of something I dreaded. As my weight went down, my self-esteem went up. I feel that I have a better quality of life now. I am finishing my freshman year in high school. I have had a great first year in high school because of learning to take better care of my body. I have been involved in several things in high school that I feel I wouldn't have been able to had I not made the change in my life. I played on the volleyball team, ran on the track team, and danced with friends in dance lessons. I have a better time with my friends now because I know that I am looking the best I can by taking care of my body. The best part is my new wardrobe!

I have learned that my Heavenly Father gave me a body to take care of and treat with respect. I am not a size 4 like a lot of my friends. But I am the best I can be, and I am happy with eating healthy and exercising and looking the best that I can. This program has changed my life.

### Note

1. J. S. Carson, F. M. Burke, and L. A. Hark, eds. *Cardiovascular Nutrition–Disease Management and Prevention* (The American Dietetic Association, 204), 177.

# Index

# Index

# Index

Percent daily value, 30
Physical conditioning, 17
Pickford, Mary, on failure, 108
Pill, 81–82
Planning, meals, 127–29, 148–224
Plant-based foods, 38–39. *See also* Specific entries for plant-based foods
Playing, as exercise, 114
Polyunsaturated fat, 52–53
Portion size. *See* Serving size
Principle, Word of Wisdom as, 5
Progression, 88–89
Protein, 9, 61–67
Prudence, definition of term, 7
Purified water, 104

Questions and answer, 203–8

Recipes, 181–98
Refrigeration, 8
Relapse, 108
Rep, 93
Resistance training, 89–96
Rest time, 93
Restaurants, 74–77, 199–202

Salad bar, 76–77
Saturated fat, 52
Seasons, for meat, 8
Self-mastery, 16–17
Serving size, 29–30, 31–38
Set, 93
Sleep, Brigham Young on, 6
Small steps, 15
Smith, Joseph Fielding, on Word of Wisdom, 5
Snacks, 100 calorie, 36–37
Social enjoyment, Brigham Young on, 6
Soreness, 92, 115
Sparingly, definition of term, 8
Sparkling water, 104–5
Spirit: making lifestyle choices through, 5; mind and body and, 16–18
Sports drinks, 103

"Spot training," 91
Spring water, 104
Stability ball, 112
Strength training, 89–96, 129–33, 162–80
Sucralose, 140
Sugar, 139–40. *See also* Artificial sweeteners
Swimming, Joseph Anderson and, 17

Target heart rate, 88
Temple, body as, 82
Testimonials, 208–24
Thirst, 101
Trans fat, 53–54
Travel, exercise and, 115–16
Treadmills, 112
Triglycerides, 54–55
TV, as exercise motivator, 114

Urine, 101

Variety, in exercise, 114–15
Veganism, 67–68
Vegetables, 6–8, 41–44
Vegetarianism, 8, 67–68
Vitamins, 140–41

Walking, strength training and, 91–92
Water. *See also* Sports drinks
Weight: disease and, 14–15; lifting, too quickly, 92–93
Weight chart, 22
Weight loss, role of calories and exercise in, 23
Wholesome herbs, 6–8
Willet, Walter, on protecting long-term health, 14
Winter, as season for meat, 8
Women, weight training and, 90
Word of Wisdom: health and, 3, 4–6; Ezra Taft Benson on wholesome living and, 10

Young, Brigham: on food, sleep, and social enjoyment, 6; on Americans' eating habits, 26; on exercise, 82; on water, 99

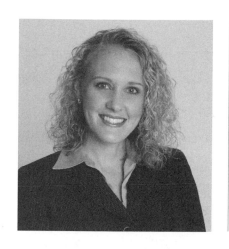

# About the Author

Melanie Douglass is a registered dietitian, a National Academy of Sports Medicine (NASM) certified personal trainer, an AFAA certified group fitness instructor, and an employee of ICON Health & Fitness. Melanie has worked in the fitness and health industry for more than 10 years, working as a weight-management consultant, clinical dietitian, and motivational speaker. She has traveled nationally to promote fitness education and has designed and appeared in several workout videos. She was recognized by the American Dietetic Association as an "Industry Mover" for her work in developing innovative fitness and nutrition programs for the consumer market. Melanie is the second counselor in the Young Women's presidency in her home ward. Melanie is the mother of three young children. Melanie and her husband Danny live in Newton, Utah.

## About ICON Health & Fitness

With approximately 3,200 employees and 11 locations around the globe, ICON Health & Fitness is one of the world's largest manufacturers and marketers of fitness equipment. ICON owns and manufactures many of the best-known brands in the fitness industry, including ProForm®, NordicTrack®, Image®, iFIT Solutions, Weider®, and HealthRider®, and licenses the popular Reebok® and Gold's Gym® brands. These brand names are immediately recognizable to consumers and have a strong reputation for high performance around the globe. ICON's commercial division, FreeMotion Fitness™, is committed to making products of unmatched quality and performance and offers the first full circuit of integrated functional training equipment, a complete line of strength-training and cardio equipment, and professional studio products for health clubs and training facilities.

ICON has consistently pioneered fitness innovation and has demonstrated its power as an industry leader by delivering state-of-the-art equipment for more than 25 years. As one of the first U.S. fitness companies to venture into the international arena, ICON has facilities in China, Europe, Canada, and the United States. No other company provides a greater selection of fitness solutions.